Studies in Systems, Decision and Control

Volume 172

The series "Studies in Systems, Decision and Control" (SSDC) covers both new developments and advances, as well as the state of the art, in the various areas of broadly perceived systems, decision making and control–quickly, up to date and with a high quality. The intent is to cover the theory, applications, and perspectives on the state of the art and future developments relevant to systems, decision making, control, complex processes and related areas, as embedded in the fields of engineering, computer science, physics, economics, social and life sciences, as well as the paradigms and methodologies behind them. The series contains monographs, textbooks, lecture notes and edited volumes in systems, decision making and control spanning the areas of Cyber-Physical Systems, Autonomous Systems, Sensor Networks, Control Systems, Energy Systems, Automotive Systems, Biological Systems, Vehicular Networking and Connected Vehicles, Aerospace Systems, Automation, Manufacturing, Smart Grids, Nonlinear Systems, Power Systems, Robotics, Social Systems, Economic Systems and other. Of particular value to both the contributors and the readership are the short publication timeframe and the world-wide distribution and exposure which enable both a wide and rapid dissemination of research output.

More information about this series at http://www.springer.com/series/13304

Salman Ben Zayed · Abdullah Bin Gani
Mohd Khalit Bin Othman

System Reengineering in Healthcare: Application for Hospital Emergency Departments

Springer

Salman Ben Zayed
Department of Computer System
and Technology, Faculty of Computer
Science and Information Technology
University of Malaya
Kuala Lumpur, Malaysia

Mohd Khalit Bin Othman
Department of Information Systems,
Faculty of Computer Science
and Information Technology
University of Malaya
Kuala Lumpur, Malaysia

Abdullah Bin Gani
Department of Computer System
and Technology, Faculty of Computer
Science and Information Technology,
Centre for Mobile Cloud Computing
Research
University of Malaya
Kuala Lumpur, Malaysia

ISSN 2198-4182 ISSN 2198-4190 (electronic)
Studies in Systems, Decision and Control
ISBN 978-3-030-07451-7 ISBN 978-3-319-98104-8 (eBook)
https://doi.org/10.1007/978-3-319-98104-8

This Springer imprint is published by the registered company Springer Nature Switzerland AG
The registered company address is: Gewerbestrasse 11, 6330 Cham, Switzerland

System Reenginering in Healthcare: Application for Hospital Emergency Departments

By

Salman Ben Zayed, Abdullah Bin Gani and
Mohd Khalid Bin Othman

Science and technology is not given, It was made by people like us. If it is not doing for us what we want, we have a right and responsibility to change it. We need a clear view of what we want for science and technology and courage to stand up and do something abut it.

Mike Cooley

To all of our families, Thank you Kindly

To all of our friends and to our faculty and university, Cant thank you enough.

Preface

This book covers an advance systematic mapping review (SMR) and state of the art taxonomy of Emergency Departments (EDs). In endeavouring to create a better understanding of the problems, methods and solutions used by experts on the topic. The authors examined previous and current research published and non-published; Journal articles, research paper, conference papers and thesis/dissertations from 1964 to 2018. The book focuses on the patient's fulfilment and how it can be enhanced. It examines existing problems like waiting time and overcrowding and how such conditions may be alleviated to provide a better service to the patients during normal and hazard mode

Six research questions were developed and was organised by advance mapping methodology and text data mining, the primary objectives for which were firstly, to obtain a common understanding of problems that need to be highlighted in EDs, and secondly, to re-analyze the methods and solutions used in available studies. The examination used in the book concentrates on quality and therefore encourages citation from important and quality source of information concerning EDs in industrial methods which can improve quality services. Various thematic areas, present in the healthcare segment, were examined through different research papers like the determination of relative efficiency and effectiveness of admission and discharge interventions; the analysis of care and managing common indications; using e-Health for enhancing effectiveness and proficiency; the seriousness of patient differences among EDs; the identification of quality problems in healthcare contexts; existing chances and the suggested plans. The book concludes that an analytical decision-making process in real-time should be used to assess a health care delivery based on its performance and KPIs modelled in this book.

It stresses the importance of deploying designed model as analytical system as modelling processes are not only important for managing patient but healthcare workforce communications but hence patient care systems as a hole. The study accounts for patient satisfaction and methods to augment it. It concentrates on satisfying the patient through reduced waiting time along with tackling issues like over congested emergency rooms so as to refine the services provided to the patients.

Furthermore, while various studies have been performed on mathematical models in general, there is a paucity of research relating to mathematical models in EDs. These kinds of studies are critical for decreasing wait times in EDs. Because healthcare systems in developing countries are very poor it is vital that issues are addressed, and requirements fulfilled for critical hospital-based healthcare. Solutions include continuous training and simulations along with comprehensive information analysis. We require a better way with the utilization of a structure, framework, process and outcomes of scientific classification to determine existing obstacles to the adoption of new model. Finally, a greater number of doctors should perform their job as doctors, instead of managing any tasks or procedures within the healthcare. A variety of research papers were investigated to address the customary scenarios in healthcare facilities such as employing e-health and mHealth for optimum effectiveness of services. The mathematical models are rarely analysed in reference to EDs; however, they are generally assessed more commonly. These studies will therefore prove advantageous for reducing waiting times in EDs and can be applied in other government agencies services as outcomes feedback tool for first time.

Kuala Lumpur, Malaysia
July 2018

Salman Ben Zayed
Abdullah Bin Gani
Mohd Khalit Bin Othman

Acknowledgements

The first edition of this book had been put together with a great deal of time and efforts from many people. Very special thanks go to both joint authors for guidance, encouragements and advices and support during one-year journey to get this book in current look and feel. This book is part of Ph.D. thesis of leading author under the supervision of both joint authors never published before elsewhere.

Kuala Lumpur, Malaysia

Salman Ben Zayed
Abdullah Bin Gani
Mohd Khalit Bin Othman

Contents

1 Background 1

2 Method 5
- 2.1 Research Questions (R.Qs) 5
- 2.2 Primary Studies Search 6
- 2.3 Study Selection 7
- 2.4 Data Extraction 8
- 2.5 Verification and Validation 8

3 Results 9
- 3.1 RQ1: Which Techniques Were Used in the ED Research? 33
- 3.2 RQ2: Which Themes Were Introduced in the ED Research? 33
- 3.3 RQ3: When and Where Was the Research Published? 34
- 3.4 RQ4: How Did the Research Illustrate the Results? 34
- 3.5 RQ5: What Problems Were Addressed in the Research? 34
- 3.6 RQ6: How Was the Research Classified? 35

4 Discussion 39

5 Conclusion and Future Research Directions 49
- 5.1 Conclusion 49
- 5.2 Future Research Direction 50

References 51

About the Authors 55

Abbreviations

ABF	Activity-Based Funding
ACR	Ambulance Call Record
ANN	Artificial Neural Network
ATS	Australian Triage Scale
CCI	The Charlson Comorbidity Index
CTAS	Canadian Emergency Departments Triage and Acuity Scale
EBP	Evidence-Based Practice
EDs	Emergency Departments
EMS	Emergency Medical Services
ESI	Emergency Severity Index
ICD	International Classification of Diseases
IEEE	Institute of Electrical and Electronics Engineers
IPO	Input-Process-Output
LOS	Length-of-Stay
LWBS	Left-Without-Being-Seen
MAC Layer	Media Access Control (Data Link)
NPs	Nurse Practitioners
PIA	Physician Initial Assessment
POF	Patient outcome feedback
QI	Quality Index
QIPS	Quality Improvement and Patient Safety
RQ.s	Research Questions
SAE	Serious Adverse Event
SLR	Systematic Literature Review
SMR	Systematic Mapping Review
TQM	Total quality Management
UST	Unified System Theory

Definitions

Dynamic Capabilities The Lean Six Sigma is widely recognized as a TQM concept which employs service engineering to conduct process redesign initiatives and efficient process management systems. These systems are beneficial in the IT departments. They utilize these systems to refabricate or automate the processes. The organizational performance can immensely benefit and conquer positive milestones from the PDCs (Process Oriented Dynamic Capabilities) that the system engages.

Process Modelling Computers are used to conduct Input Process Output (IPO). The process should have enough room for specific adjustments so that the employs can tailor fit it to their requirements. Uncertainties are likely to occur therefore the employees must take efficiency into account when modelling new systems.

Service Engineering During the process, the services are developed and modified along each production unit. Services are typically a process but have been widely considered as a product. The service world requires a unified theory to be presented with so as to efficiently engage the services. For this purpose, the Unified service theory (UST) is brought to service through the I/O process model. An appropriate technique for transitioning input into output is only possible when the I/O model is analysed in the light of certain features.

Simulation Method Organizations are applying a wide variety of simulation methods. The discrete-event—simulation is the primary method that is used for the modelling of a company's operation systems—queening systems.

Simulation Model There are various complex computer models present but the simulation method can be used as a real-world phenomenon to establish a model that would help study the target simply rather than actually studying the target.

Utilization To bring something to use in its optimum capacity is known as utilization. This includes evaluating daily tangible assets, equipment, proceeds and success rate of workload and acquired milestones.

Optimization A real function can be capitalized or diminished by making calculated choices between pre-determined ranges of input values. The optimum value of the function is achieved through the substituting from the range of alternate values offered.

Emergency Preparedness Is collective actions for immediate relief and hazardous effective operation management before, during and after force of nature, human actions including a plan will help with safety, security and comfort regardless disaster type. In other words, it's a strategy for risk reduction before, during and after crises for known capacity that requires the necessary tools and steps to assess hazards; it must be followed by vulnerable resources and work and activities of people at local, regional and national level in which need development and strengthening services of emergency in form of large scale emergency, disaster response and relief or recovery program.

Management The capacity to recognize complicated issues to forecast disasters/hazardous with appropriate knowledge is related with the effective recognition of change, employing relative programs, calculating the operational efficiency in application to assess possible malfunctions in the system in other words, identifying change, utilizing strategies, evaluating the operational capacity in real world.

Emergency Departments Is a system of people (patients, healthcare workforce, engineers and administrative staff) including processes and medical advancement and technologies in forms of hardware and software connected together with a network (cables, Wi-Fi, etc) to produce outputs that's is immediate quality care in other words, The production of outputs with the help of network of hardware and software, like cables, Wi-Fi etc.

List of Figures

Fig. 1.1 Simulation modeling kind utilized from 2000–2009 2
Fig. 1.2 Countries using the simulation model in hazard mode 2006–2012 2
Fig. 1.3 Data collection types in simulation model at normal mode. 3
Fig. 1.4 Data collection types in simulation model at hazard mode 3
Fig. 2.1 Study selection process. 7
Fig. 3.1 Subjects with a research gap in performance measurement. 35
Fig. 3.2 Overview of topics with research gaps (emergency preparedness and quality of healthcare) 35
Fig. 3.3 Where the studies were published. 36
Fig. 3.4 When the studies were published 36
Fig. 3.5 Classification of studies. 37
Fig. 3.6 Thematic studies cluster 37
Fig. 4.1 Quality clusters in healthcare 40
Fig. 4.2 Input-process-output (IPO) model. 40
Fig. 4.3 EDs operational management cluster. 42
Fig. 4.4 Workforce clusters in healthcare 43
Fig. 4.5 Healthcare workforce performance model. 44
Fig. 4.6 Emergency preparedness clusters in healthcare 45
Fig. 4.7 Quality engineering clusters in healthcare. 45
Fig. 4.8 Utilization clusters in healthcare 46
Fig. 4.9 Simulation clusters in healthcare. 47

List of Tables

Table 1.1 Simulation model in normal mode 1974–2015 2
Table 2.1 Database searches and results 6
Table 2.2 Revised data extraction table 8
Table 3.1 Quality care: general and current concerns 10
Table 3.2 EDs operational management 13
Table 3.3 Healthcare workforce 21
Table 3.4 Emergency preparedness 23
Table 3.5 Quality engineering 25
Table 3.6 Utilization in healthcare 27
Table 3.7 Simulation in healthcare 29
Table 3.8 Thematic clusters with references 37

Abstract

Emergency departments (EDs) provide vital services that involve complex systems to ensure that patients are treated appropriately. Treatment choices are made based on real-time data. However, it would facilitate the prediction of the failure of a patient's treatment through in-depth manual examinations and the evaluation of problems that are related to the effective management of operations. This book explores previous mapping studies that use effective reviews as evidence. The use of reengineering systems and the quality assessment of the healthcare model, especially in the hazard mode, plays an important role in determining patients' satisfaction and the effects of operational management on patients' understanding. This book presents a systematic review and taxonomy of previous research published from 1964 to 2018 on the management and operation of EDs. The purpose of our book is to create a better understanding of the methods, problems and solutions used by experts during the study period by focusing on patient satisfaction in normal and hazard boundary settings in optimal quality healthcare operation management particularly in research published within the last decade.

Keywords Emergency department · Quality · Healthcare · Management
Emergency preparedness · Systematic review · Skills and competencies
Real-time algorithm · Patient satisfaction · Utilization and simulation

Introduction

The present investigation of previous studies according to their taxonomy and input consisted of searching for the available literature [1], examining it, and recognizing particular patterns and similarities among the research techniques and the publications. Emergency departments (EDs) are capable of responding to different kinds of intense emergencies by providing critical emergency care both in and outside the hospital. A decision-analytical model is required to evaluate health operations. These processes are required to be updated by hospitals because the communications between patients and ED staff as well as patient care pathways and monitoring are conducted by applying modelling techniques. Because of the complex nature of EDs and the different problems faced by them, it is important to examine the system. Although mathematical models of healthcare have been used in previous research, such models have been rarely used in the research on EDs. Nevertheless, such models play a significant part in minimizing the extensive waiting times experienced in EDs.

In the healthcare business, primarily in emergency medical departments in underdeveloped countries, the enhancement of facilities and quality measurements has proven highly useful in evaluating the quality and success of the treatment services offered to patients. Such evaluations include the viewpoint of other patients. From a logical perspective, it is not simple to recognize a definite conceptual measurement of facilities in EDs. The available monitoring and operation techniques used to measure service quality are not used by the EDs in these countries. From a technological perspective, the aspects leading to the effective establishment of an e-quality observational system for emergency medical services can be used as archetypes.

Several intricate aspects are involved in carrying out the operational management of an emergency. It is very important to adopt efficient methods to ensure that patients receive quick responses to their queries. Emergency preparedness has been a highly recorded issue in EDs regarding extensive waiting periods and overcrowding, particularly during disasters. Overcrowding is associated with higher fatality and readmission rates, the higher probability of patients' leaving without being seen. Moreover, there is a higher incidence of inappropriate services for patients because of the need to prioritize the treatment of a huge volume of patients whose symptoms can range from the trivial to the acute. The procedure begins with the patient's admission to the hospital, monitoring by a doctor and then treatment with the proper medical care.

A gap in the knowledge was recognized. The selected topics were divided according to the EDs, and mapping was conducted on 1,241,530 articles that were published from 1964 to 2018. The research approaches in [2] and [3] were utilized. The research questions were formulated based on the activities of EDs. The major issues in the EDs and the techniques used by them were categorized. The findings showed several inadequacies in the healthcare business, such as emergency preparedness, quality of healthcare and performance assessment. The implementation of procedures based on these findings could influence not only ED systems but also entire institutions that pursue excellence in service, such as the healthcare industry and e-government systems.

Chapter 1
Background

A simple structure for real-world implementation is offered by the mathematical modeling methods that are used to plan industrial engineering and operational procedures. Although EDs do not have unlimited means, they offer critical treatment to a huge percentage of the patient population. The assessment of ED systems involves the examination of resource consumption, quantity, and waiting times.

In the case of extensive waiting times, overcrowding can occur in EDs, which can result in the increased risk of patient death. Furthermore, patients may depart without being seen, which leads to their readmission to EDs. It is important to consider the organizational, physical, and human aspects of patient monitoring in ED environments. Hence, the operational management system, equipment, buildings, real-time information about patients and their families must also be considered. Primary prerequisites are waiting areas and other areas where overcrowding is prohibited during the hours of highest risk. Patients are managed according to the following guidelines: listing the name of the patient, triage, inspection, x-rays, blood tests, assessment, pharmacy, ED bed location, ED staff, management, allocation, and finally discharge.

Overcrowding can result in an increased waiting times in the ED. Furthermore, the capacity may not be sufficient to fulfill the requirements. There might not be enough beds, capacity management might not be effective, and patient acuteness and service requirements may differ [4]. The discrete-event simulation technique was considered the most widespread technique utilized in EDs, particularly in the UK Healthcare system from 2000–2009 [4]. System dynamics has been used to some extent to reduce the waiting times in EDs (Fig. 1.1).

Because EDs aim to achieve significant healthcare goals, they are perceived as the most vital component in the hospital. EDs are required to formulate logical solutions and processes in both normal and adverse circumstances. Problems that pertain to prevention, minimizing waiting times, predicting variables in normal and adverse circumstances in EDs can be addressed by simulation software. Problems that take place in real settings as well as issues related to patient flow and monitoring, arrival patterns, and irregular withdrawal of optimal means in emergency response areas [5] are determined by the simulation model (Table 1.1 and Fig. 1.2).

S. Ben Zayed et al., *System Reengineering in Healthcare: Application for Hospital Emergency Departments*, Studies in Systems, Decision and Control 172,
https://doi.org/10.1007/978-3-319-98104-8_1

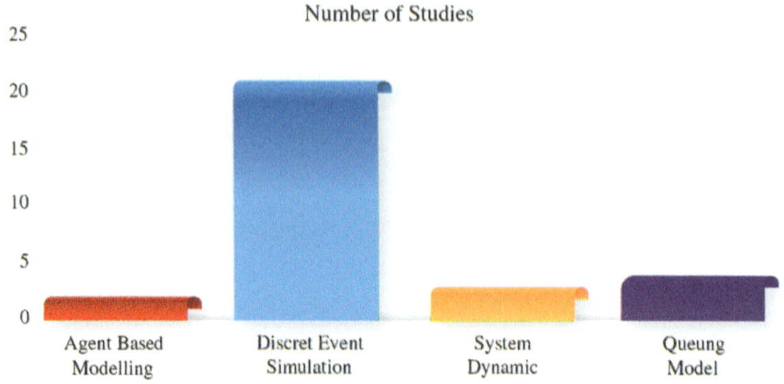

Fig. 1.1 Simulation modeling kind utilized from 2000–2009

Table 1.1 Simulation model in normal mode 1974–2015

USA	49%	Israel	2%
UK	14%	Ireland	2%
Turkey	1%	Iran	3%
Taiwan	3%	Hong Kong	1%
Sweden	1%	Germany	1%
Spain	3%	France	2%
Singapore	2%	Finland	1%
Norway	2%	Chile	1%
Kuwait	1%	Canada	5%
Jordan	2%	Australia	1%
Italy	2%	Total	100%

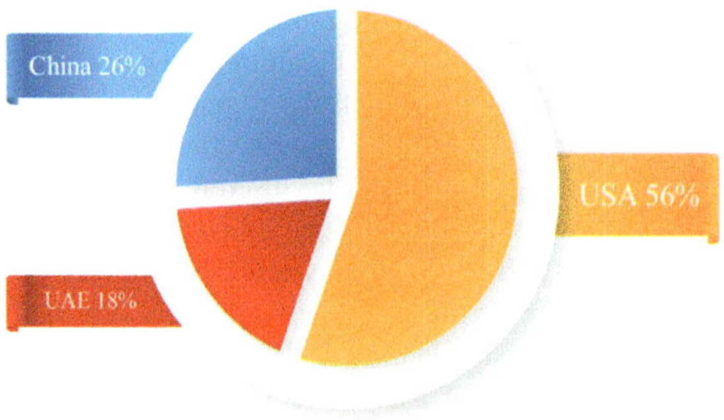

Fig. 1.2 Countries using the simulation model in hazard mode 2006–2012

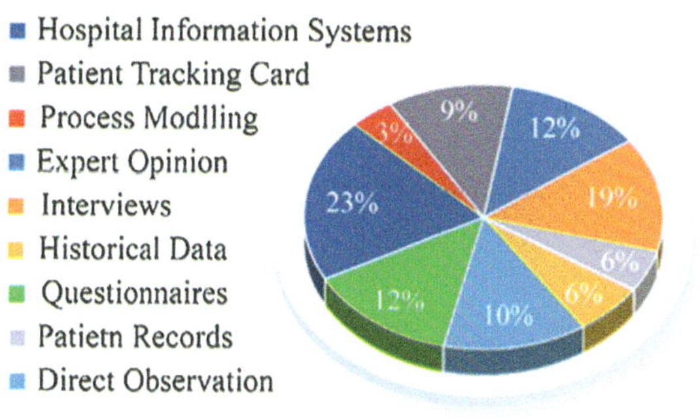

Fig. 1.3 Data collection types in simulation model at normal mode

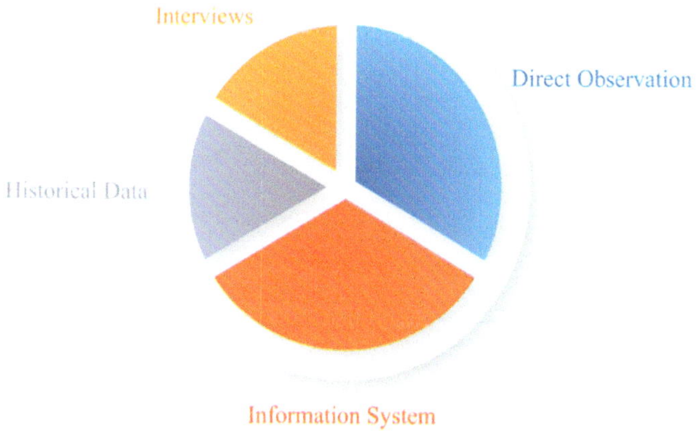

Fig. 1.4 Data collection types in simulation model at hazard mode

In the simulation model, data are collected differently in normal and risky modes. Data are collected from direct sampling, historical data, hospital databases, question naires, patient tracking cards, and observations (Figs. 1.3 and 1.4). Simulation techniques are implemented to improve resources and minimize waiting times through the application of cost scrutinization and the presentation of planned policies [5].

Chapter 2
Method

Information that is up-to-date is highly helpful. Representing a system, or systematic mapping, is the preliminary step in assessing the available literature according to subject and classifying it in order to carry out a thematic assessment. This research offers detailed descriptions of previous studies. Overviews of the research area and the research limitations are offered by the systematic mapping paper. This research uses the latest sources. Systematic mapping enables researchers to analyze research papers based on a particular subject [6] and categorize them in order to carry out a thematic assessment. The available research examined using a systematic review procedure that follows a definite protocol [7]. Hence, the aim of a mapping study is to specify the research area and differentiate the limitations of previous studies.

2.1 Research Questions (R.Qs)

In this systematic review, the observational approaches in [1–3] were used to identify the issues encountered in EDs. Based on these issues, six research questions were developed:

- RQ1: Which methods were utilized in the ED research?
- RQ2: What themes were introduced in the ED research?
- RQ3: When and where was the research published?
- RQ4: How did the research illustrate the results?
- RQ5: What issues were addressed in the research? What were the findings?
- RQ6: How was the research categorized?

We organized our research based on the results of the mapping study. The research questions were used to guide the methodology of our research. The following are the primary objectives of our study: (a) to gain a common understanding of the problems that need to be highlighted in EDs and (b) to re-analyze the methods used in the available studies.

S. Ben Zayed et al., *System Reengineering in Healthcare: Application for Hospital Emergency Departments*, Studies in Systems, Decision and Control 172,
https://doi.org/10.1007/978-3-319-98104-8_2

2.2 Primary Studies Search

The research was conducted in the following databases: ABI/INFORM [8–13], Annual Reviews [14–20], Bio One [21], Cambridge Journal Online [22–44], Emerald [45, 46], IEEE Xplore [47–51], ProQuest Dissertations & Theses Global [52–57], and IoP Science Journal [58–62]. These databases were selected because they are considered the largest databases of millions of periodicals about EDs, engineering, and computer science. Furthermore, these databases are easy to use because they have excellent search features. The following keywords were used: emergency department, emergency medical care, emergency clinics, and methods. The subsequent search strings were created by using these keywords:

- Set1: Search terms regarding scoping research on EDs (i.e., *emergency department*)
- Set2: Search terms regarding the string (e.g. *emergency medical care* and *emergency clinics*)
- Set3: Search terms regarding approaches (e.g., *methods*).

Table 2.1 Database searches and results

Database	Command search	All results	Results from 2010–2018	Final results 2010–2018
ABI/INFORM	("emergency department" or "emergency medical care" or "emergency clinics") and ("methods")	103,025 (1864–2017)	11,232	6
Emerald		12,313 (1898–2017)	966	2
IEEE Xplore		891 (1929–2017)	641	5
ProQuest Dissertations		265,631 (1897–2017)	56,901	6
Annual Reviews		13,060 (2007–2017)	10,273	7
Bio One		391 (2001–2017)	200	1
Cambridge Journals Online		846,098 (1900–2017)	1384	23
IoP Science Journal		121 (1980–2017)	68	5
Total		1,241,530 (1864–2017)	81,665	55

The keywords were categorized according to the research questions and then divided into three sets. The database yielded every set. All the search strings are shown in Table 2.1. This research was conducted in early 2018. The number of search findings from each database is shown in Table 2.1.

2.3 Study Selection

The items that included numerous database features were overlooked (Fig. 2.1). The initial quality assessment focused on the citations in each article. Some articles without citations were not included. Studies were included based on the following criteria: studies that concentrated on research techniques used to analyze EDs; studies published between 2010 and 2018; and studies on EDs. Some studies then were excluded based on the following criteria: studies not in full text form; studies that were not reviewed; studies that were copied other research; studies in languages other than English. Figure 2.1 represents the number of articles that were included and excluded as a result of the database search. The final selection is shown in Tables 3.1–3.7.

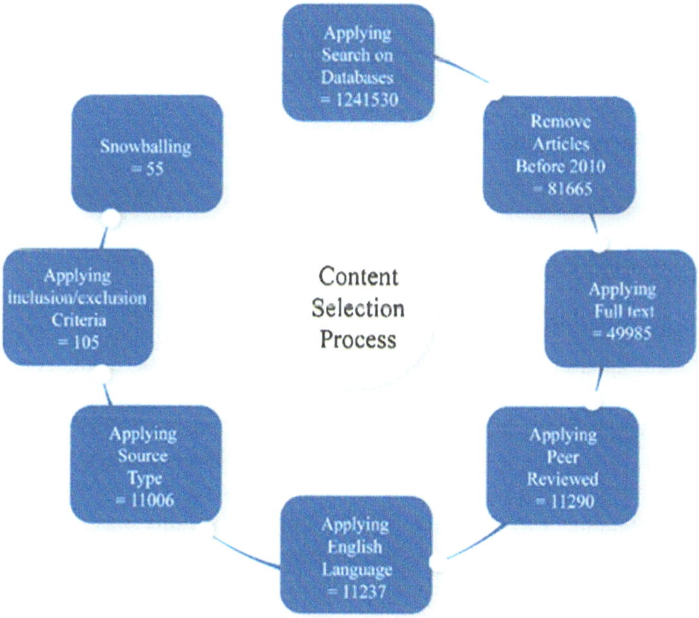

Fig. 2.1 Study selection process

Table 2.2 Revised data extraction table

Item	RQ result	RQ
Author name	Name(s)	
Year of publication	Calendar year	RQ3
Country	Location of study	RQ3
EDs area	Knowledge area in EDs	RQ2
Venue	Journal name	RQ3
Method	Method used	RQ1
Problem/issue	Problem/objective identified	RQ5
Visualization type	Style of presentation	RQ4
Conclusion	Final result of the study	RQ5
Article type	Classification of content	RQ6

2.4 Data Extraction

The excluded data were based on the pattern presented in [3], which was adapted for this research, as shown in Table 2.2. The item and the value are shown in each data field. Data mining and abstraction were performed and examined by the first author and then assessed by the second and third authors for validity and quality control. Table 2.2 is based on six research questions. An additional examination was carried out through text mining using the NVivo [68] software to extract subjects and trees. Other relevant findings were gathered from the databases as the initial findings of the first mapping procedure.

2.5 Verification and Validation

The gathered data were highly objective. This type of validity is less risky than the data gathered using quantitative methods. To further reduce the risk, a data compilation table was used to support the documented data. The data mining table in [2] was adapted to enable the re-analysis. Data mining tables are used to record data and minimize risk. Moreover, it is possible to review the data extraction by which risk can also be minimized. These steps were conducted separately by two authors. A shared understanding was achieved, and the threat to validity was minimized [3]. The data collected in this research were precise and impartial; therefore, the degree of risk was minimized [1–3] and [6, 7].

Chapter 3
Results

In every database [8–59], numerous publications were recognized and revised between 2010 and 2017. Other relevant results are shown in Tables 3.1, 3.2, 3.3, 3.4, 3.5, 3.6 and 3.7. The research questions are addressed in Sects. 3.1–3.6. A thematic analysis was conducted, and the subjects were categorized based on the quality that led to the enhancement of the general results on EDs: Quality Care, overall and existing apprehension; EDs Operational Administration; Healthcare Staff Abilities and Attuited; Emergency Preparedness; Quality Engineering; Utilization in Healthcare; Simulation in Healthcare. We developed the tables according to the seven themes that emerged from the cluster result examination instead of only one table consisting of the 55 selected articles. We began with Table 3.1 and ended with Table 3.7.

The examination used in the book concentrates on quality and therefore encourages citations of important situations concerning EDs in experimental methods that can improve quality services. Many of the research outcomes in the health segment were represented by the use of object clusters and the association with uncertain qualities. The major aspects that were discovered in the quality of the delivery of healthcare services and the relevant study results were found in the research data published in the USA [14, 18] and Canada. The important aspects concerning quality were as follows: performance [26], improvement procedures [36], and decision-making [31] in EDs. The important debate in this book was based on the analytical method that is used in improving operational management specifically in the healthcare segment in the EDs. This research employed both qualitative and quantitative techniques of evidence-based practice [31] and item perceiving. As per the general perspective, a combination of different methods was used. However, in majority of situations, qualitative and quantitative methods were employed.

Various themes in the healthcare segment were examined in several studies, such as the determination of the relative efficiency of pre-discharge [13] interventions, the analysis of the care and management of common indications [14] during the last stages of life, and the use of e-Health [18] to enhance effectiveness [36] and proficiency. The seriousness of patient differences among EDs was examined. Moreover, quality problems and opportunities in healthcare contexts were identified, and plans

S. Ben Zayed et al., *System Reengineering in Healthcare: Application for Hospital Emergency Departments*, Studies in Systems, Decision and Control 172,
https://doi.org/10.1007/978-3-319-98104-8_3

Table 3.1 Quality care: general and current concerns

Author and year	Country	Extracted data
Scott, 2010	Australia	**Area in EDs**: Quality: procedures of hospital discharge. **Location**: Australian Health Review. **Methodology**: Qualitative: analysis and Systematic meta-analysis of controlled trials. **Problem/Issue**: To identify the comparative proficiency of per discharge interferences prior to or after the discharge. **Visualization Kind**: Text: Percentages and categorizations plus table. **Conclusion**: Most of single-factor interferences, which fail to cover the hospital municipal boundary appear as less efficient in decreasing the readmission rate as compared to the multifactor interferences directed at increased-risk populations involving pre- and post-discharge features. **Publication Kind**: Journal Article
Abrahm, 2011	United States	**Area in EDs**: Quality: Management—Common Signs. **Location**: Annual Report of Medicine. **Methodology**: Mixed techniques: Evaluation Technique and scoring with forms. **Problem/Issue**: To examine the care and organization of common sign taking place during End of Life. **Visualization Kind**: Forms. **Conclusion**: The Centre to Advance Palliative Care has played an important role in the quick growth and maintenance of agendas concerning palliative care in the United States. Palliative care programs are being carried out in 70% of hospitals having >200 beds. **Publication Kind**: Journal Article
Meier et al., 2013	United States	**Area in EDs**: Quality: eHealth and Effectiveness; Record keeping and Cloud Computing. **Location**: Annual Review Biomedical Engineering. **Methodology**: Qualitative: systematic review. **Problem/Issue**: To keep the record of the history of eHealth and to assure the consumption of Internet-based information technology (IT) in order to affectedly enhance the effectiveness of health-care services provision. **Visualization Kind**: Figures, Tables and Charts. **Conclusion**: The increasing rate of Healthcare is not viable anymore in the developed states, since demographics, age structures, and lifestyles are constantly changing. **Publication Kind**: Journal Article

(continued)

Table 3.1 (continued)

Author and year	Country	Extracted data
Cheung et al., 2016	Canada	**Area in EDs**: Quality: Performance Evaluation and Record Keeping. **Location**: Canadian Journal of Emergency Medicine. **Methodology**: Quantitative: Daily Clinical Evaluation Report Rating. Linear regression analysis was used in order to evaluate an alternative measure of resident performance. **Problem/Issue**: To distinguish the value of high quality work-related evaluations achieved. **Visualization Kind**: Graphs. **Conclusion**: The quality of recorded clinical performance evaluations with 9 items tool are influenced by the inhabitant performance and trainee vicinity. **Publication Kind**: Journal Article
Grafstein et al., 2016	Canada	**Area in EDs**: Quality: Administration (Patients categorization and diagnosis and Standards CCI and ICD. **Location**: Canadian Journal of Emergency Medicine. **Methodology**: Quantitative: local data 2.5-year period. **Problem/Issue**: To estimate the seriousness of patient's condition and differences among Eds for the administration of same situations depending on the International Classification of Diseases (ICD) diagnosis codes. **Visualization Kind**: Tables. **Conclusion**: In over-all 11 EDs (involving 6 urban and 5 rural areas), 931,596 local ED visits were made by 446,579 different patients. The Charlson Comorbidity Index (CCI) is a new technique through which inactively patient comorbidities can be recorded inactively without depending on a data entry expert. **Publication Kind**: Journal Article
Jensen et al., 2016	Canada	**Area in EDs**: Quality: Procedure Enhancement, Abilities and Aptitudes and Decision Making. **Location**: Canadian Association of Emergency Physicians. **Methodology**: Evidence based practice (EBP), clinical practice rules/ code of behaviour, by means of a recognized approach. **Problem/Issue**: To identify the available chances and offer consistent suggested plans for regional and national EMS organizations for enhancing patient health results, the competence and quality of EMS systems of care, and security of patients and EMS experts. **Visualization Kind**: Charts, Figures, and tables. **Conclusion**: In order to enhance the results, involving clinical system, safety, and quality. Canadian EDs services will use the best accessible proof. **Publication Kind**: Journal Article

(continued)

Table 3.1 (continued)

Author and year	Country	Extracted data
Leung et al., 2017a	Canada	**Area in EDs**: Quality: Process development and process reengineering; operational influence on patient flow management, LOS and effectiveness. **Location**: Canadian Journal of Emergency Medicine. **Methodology**: Quantitative: restructuring triage, comparable processing, adjustable nurse-patient proportions, flexible exam seats, and adjustable physician planning were included in Segmented regression for chart analysis for 36-month at an urban community emergency department from January 2010 to December 2012. **Problem/Issue**: To analyse the operational effects of an interference consisting of concurrent procedure enhancements to triage, patient entry, and physician planning arrangements on emergency department (ED) patient flow. Any rise in ED resources or expenses was not obliged by the interference. **Visualization Kind**: Tables and Charts. **Conclusion**: The ED was joined by 251,899 patients during their studies. A sequence of process enhancements intended to improve flow in the ED without adding resources was linked with clinically noteworthy declines in length of stay (LOS), physician initial assessment (PIA), left-without-being-seen (LWBS) and left-against-medical-advice (LAMA) degrees for non-resuscitative patients. **Publication Kind**: Journal Article
Buttigieg et al., 2016	Malta	**Area in EDs**: Quality: Continuous Quality Improvement, Process Reengineering, and strategic management. **Location**: Journal of Health Organization and Management. **Methodology**: Multiple case study methodology: efficient strategic planning and project management methodology: suggested technique to three units. **Problem/Issue**: To determine the way in which the logical framework analysis could be used to offer and form cases in the healthcare field. **Visualization Kind**: Tables, Figures and Charts. **Conclusion**: The ageing population is an important challenge, which is leading to an augmented requirement for health facilities along with lengthy waiting lists for severe services, restoration therapies and long-term care. **Publication Kind**: Research Paper

Table 3.2 EDs operational management

Author and year	Country	Extracted data
Hanson, 2011	Australia	**Area in EDs**: Management strategies. **Location**: Australian Health Review Methodology: **Problem/Issue**: To show that a structured strategy is required by healthcare systems to improve data quality and an attempt to establish a vigorous information system. **Visualization Kind**: Process. **Conclusion**: Controlling healthcare workforce abilities through the available information, guaranteeing all departments were sustained, founding a platform, maintaining liability at the department level, refining system competence and performance, determining, and restructuring data flow streams to guarantee relevance for all patients by involving all patient settings in all facilities. **Publication Kind**: Journal Article
Baicker et al., 2012	United States	**Area in EDs**: Management: cost and expenses. **Location**: Annual Review of Economics. **Methodology**: Quantitative analysis: local differences of insurance payments and salaries, health expenses, Healthcare costs. **Problem/Issue**: To assess allocative effectiveness and to make a comparison between the spending and results in various geographic parts to determine the degree of improvements in results that accumulate to greater spending and then to compare those to output in other areas. **Visualization Kind**: Tables and Graphs. **Conclusion**: Healthcare systems should be established to stimulate that intervention and encourage its consumption in patients for whom high health profits will ensue without becoming indebted to massive government subsidies to compensate its usage in patients with little to no advantage. **Publication Kind**: Journal Article
Clifford and Clifton, 2012	United States	**Area in EDs**: Management: wireless technology (mHealth). **Location**: Annual Review of Medicine. **Methodology**: Qualitative: review. **Problem/Issue**: To explain the importance of wireless technology, particularly when it is used in the management of diseases and medicine. **Visualization Kind**: Graphs. **Conclusion**: There are numerous benefits of delivering healthcare services by mHealth over current care pathways: Data are uploaded automatically, Natural track for data response, enables maintaining long-term medical records, enables in-depth modified healthcare, individual, identifier e.g., International mobile equipment identity (IMEI), natural safety, data upload within precise period, a general boundary that can be modified without any difficulty, users' acquaintance with devices, and decreased rate of capital investment. **Publication Kind**: Review Paper

(continued)

Table 3.2 (continued)

Author and year	Country	Extracted data
Kaplan et al., 2013	United States	**Area in EDs**: **Management**: Patient record: mHealth. **Location**: Annual Review of Psychology. **Methodology**: Qualitative: SMR (Tables for mHealth information technology) review. **Problem/Issue**: The study assessed the significance of mobile technologies in determining the positive behaviours, self-reports, and functional responses. It assessed interventions that used mobile technologies. More than half remained unsuccessful in recording important improvements in health results or health risk aspects. **Visualization Kind**: Graphs, Figures, and Tables. **Conclusion**: There has already been an intense influence of mobile electronic technologies on the assessments of important developments in our capability of analyzing conduct outside the laboratory. **Publication Kind**: Journal Article
Atkinson, 2016	Canada	**Area in EDs**: Management: patient experience and waiting period at EDs. **Location**: Canadian Journal of Emergency Medicine. **Methodology**: **Qualitative**: **investigation**. **Problem/Issue**: To discover the view of time in emergency medicine as perceived by both the healthcare suppliers as well as the patients and handle the ever-rising line of waiting patients. **Visualization Kind**: Figures. **Conclusion**: ED system planning should recognize the actual dangers in the time we devote profoundly to patients and guarantee that upcoming advances in management procedures do not increase such risks. **Publication Kind**: Conference Paper
Chartier et al., 2016a	Canada	**Area in EDs**: Management: EDs services (point-of-care). **Location**: Canadian Journal of Emergency Medicine. **Methodology**: Qualitative research: systematic analysis + meta review through two databases: MEDLINE and EMBASE. **Problem/Issue**: To assess the implementation of point-of-care for identifying the disease and evaluating the success rate of decrease trials. **Visualization Kind**: Charts and Tables. **Conclusion**: Avoiding additions in the meta review presented good test features for the diagnosis and the use of plain radiography at present should not be fully replaced by the decline. This evaluation showed that it is an influential assistant in all circumstances and could be consumed as a rational substitute in particular contexts. **Publication Kind**: Conference Paper

(continued)

Table 3.2 (continued)

Author and year	Country	Extracted data
Ducharme, 2016	Canada	**Area in EDs**: Management: Crowding and Healthcare Staff abilities. **Location**: Canadian Journal of Emergency Medicine. **Methodology**: Qualitative: grounded theory. **Problem/Issue**: To form an accurate system for appropriate end-of-life care involving the formation of bounds for when we will not be offering active care services anymore since crowding is an indicator of impairment and we do not require that indicator to acknowledge we want an accurate system. **Visualization Kind**: Percentages. **Conclusion**: Describing and responding to the question that has always been avoided: "Define emergency medicine, and who should be present in the emergency department?" After addressing that question for implementing emergency medicine, we would address the way in which it should be done by using the skills to treat those who really require it. **Publication Kind**: Conference Paper
Holroyd et al., 2016	Canada	**Area in EDs**: Management: Triage Level, Ordering of Patients. **Location**: Canadian Journal of Emergency Medicine. **Methodology**: Quantitative: using the National Ambulatory Care Reporting System dataset. **Problem/Issue**: To compare EDs, to define ED patient case mix, and to place ED patients in order. To determine whether or not the triage score can be used as an effective emergency department measure. The circulation of the scores of the patients were assessed by the authors on CTAS and the percentage in admission. **Visualization Kind**: Tables. **Conclusion**: Additional work is needed to precisely illustrate ED patient case mix triage system cannot be used as an exclusive technique for comparing and explaining the emergency department case mix. **Publication Kind**: Conference Paper
Imperato et al., 2017	Canada	**Area in EDs**: Management: Triage Level, Vital Signs assessments. **Location**: Canadian Journal of Emergency Medicine. **Methodology**: Experimental controlled attempt: heart rate <40 beats per minute or >130 beats per minutes, respiratory rate <8 breaths per minute or >30 breaths per minute, systolic blood pressure <90 mm Hg, or oxygen saturation $<90\%$ on room temperature. **Problem/Issue**: To determine whether the inpatient hospital metrics were measurably influenced by a clinical triggers program in the ED setting that used predefined irregular dynamic signs to trigger a quick evaluation by an emergency physician-led multidisciplinary team. **Visualization Kind**: Tables. **Conclusion**: No difference was perceived among the groups in median days spent for inpatient care (3.8 v. 4.0 days, $p=0.21$) or median days spent in a special care unit (5.0 v. 5.6 days, $p=0.42$). The percentage of in-hospital patient deaths remained the same (6.0% v. 5.6%, $p=0.66$) in addition to the rate of improvement in level of care within 24 h (4.9% v. 4.0%, $p=0.52$). It was concluded that, the application of an ED clinical triggers program did not lead to a noteworthy progress in the evaluated inpatient results. **Publication Kind**: Journal Article

(continued)

Table 3.2 (continued)

Author and year	Country	Extracted data
Krebs et al., 2016a	Canada	**Area in EDs**: Management: non-urgent presentation to ED. **Location**: Canadian Journal of Emergency Medicine. **Methodology**: Mixed: quantitative: questionnaire used (randomly chosen from electronic registration records at three city EDs). Qualitative (categorization): the answers were analyzed using a thematic content analysis by relying on past knowledge and reviewing the literature. **Problem/Issue**: To analyze the explanations provided by patients for their presentation to the ED, regardless of being recognized as "non-urgent" (CTAS 3–5). A significant discussion exists concerning the contribution of non-urgent, low acuity visits to the ED and the role they play in overcrowding. Not much is known about these low acuity presentations. **Visualization Kind**: Graphs, Figures and Tables. **Conclusion**: The research revealed that it is important to accept different reasons for emergency department presentations for applying techniques to encourage non-urgent care requirements. **Publication Kind**: Conference Paper
Krebs et al., 2016b	Canada	**Area in EDs**: Management: quality and standardized device for decisions related to care. **Location**: Canadian Journal of Emergency Medicine. **Methodology**: Quantitative: questionnaire surveys of 50 patients and 50 clinicians. **Problem/Issue**: To assess the pertinence of a tool formed by an emergency department team to reverse the corroboration this supports Choosing Wisely Canada (CWC). **Visualization Kind**: Tables and Graphs **Conclusion**: suggested that a tool should be established to help involve patients and clinicians in conversation concerning unnecessary care in the emergency departments. **Publication Kind**: Conference Paper
Leggatt et al., 2016	Canada	**Area in EDs**: Management: ACR, vital signs and record keeping. **Location**: Canadian Journal of Emergency Medicine. **Methodology**: Experiment-control group: in one year (Jan–Dec 2013), all LA calls were received by a single EMS agency, which were analyzed for absent vital-sign documentation. **Problem/Issue**: To determine whether a difference exist between Ambulance call record (ACR) documentation of vital signs and Lift Assist (LA): (In case treatment is not managed and the patient is not conveyed to hospital) calls and non-LA calls and to identify the differences among ACR keeping of the vital signs in the midst of the non-LA and LA calls conveyed to the emergency department for medical assessment. **Visualization Kind**: Tables and Charts. **Conclusion**: There were considerably more patient rejections for receiving vitals than conveyed to patients. It should be ensured that these patients are treated with the similar quality of care as well as the documentation of patients calling EMS for obvious medical issues. **Publication Kind**: Journal Article

(continued)

Table 3.2 (continued)

Author and year	Country	Extracted data
Leung et al., 2016b	Canada	**Area in EDs**: Management: use; patient flow and EDs effectiveness. **Location**: Canadian Journal of Emergency Medicine Chart. **Methodology**: Analysis for 48 months at the emergency department of an urban community from September 2011 to September 2015. 399,958 patients joined the ED in the course of the research. **Problem/Issue**: To enhance the effectiveness of emergency departments, to increase patient flow as much as possible, and to analyze how the emergency department patient flow is operationally affected by PM. Visualization Kind: Tables and Charts. Conclusion: Patient flow on a daily basis can be augmented by up to 11.2% with no major rises in the number of physicians' shifts per day or in the per day hours of physician while the post-intervention. The application of Physician Navigators is linked with the noteworthy decreases in the rates of LOS, PIA, and LWBS for non-resuscitative patients at a huge capacity emergency department. **Publication Kind**: Journal Article
MacKay et al., 2016	Canada	**Area in EDs**: Management: triage level; waiting duration and job allocation. **Location**: Canadian Journal of Emergency Medicine. **Methodology**: Quantitative: cross-sectional surveys and Descriptive statistics were measured. **Problem/Issue**: To determine the frequency of formal triage systems in PC appointment allocation. **Visualization Kind**: Tables and Charts. **Conclusion**: A formal triage system was not used in any crucial care practices to allocate appointments, regardless of extensive waiting periods, which were protracted up to 50 days. **Publication Kind**: Journal Article
Pinto and Lajoie, 2016	Canada	**Area in EDs**: Management: patient fulfilment. **Location**: Canadian Journal of Emergency Medicine. **Methodology**: Quantitative: online survey. **Problem/Issue**: To determine if emergency medicine physicians and resident clinicians looking for patient comments encountered noteworthy obstacles and to identify contemporary practices of hospital workers their behaviour in response to patient outcome feedback. **Visualization Kind**: Charts. **Conclusion**: Patient outcome feedback POF is a beneficial and vital practice for clinical care but is not frequently carried out at present in determining the kinds of patients that are considered the most pertinent for obtaining POF. The frequency with which POF is pursued can be enhanced by identifying the main hurdles encountered by clinicians, which could refine patient care. **Publication Kind**: Journal Article

(continued)

Table 3.2 (continued)

Author and year	Country	Extracted data
Sprackman et al., 2016	Canada	**Area in EDs**: Management: deficiency of communication, use, patient anticipation, knowledge administration, and access to waiting time for patient. **Location**: Canadian Journal of Emergency Medicine. **Methodology**: A two-stage combined techniques research was carried out at a dual campus tertiary care academic centre. Qualitative: focus group discussions. Quantitative: a patient survey. **Problem/Issue**: To offer an insight into patients' requirements with reference to issuing ED waiting times. This, to our knowledge, has not been mentioned in the prior literature. To build understanding of the needs of the patients regarding the publication of the emergency department waiting times, which has not been extensively explained in the prior literature. **Visualization Kind**: Table and Figures. **Conclusion**: Content analysis illustrates that: having access to information, such as waiting time, wait time posting, absence of communication, training in waiting room, patient prospects, consumption of the ED, patient conduct, physical ease, and patient authorization, greatly effects the development of understanding concerning patients' requirement. **Publication Kind**: Journal Article
VandenBerg et al., 2016	Canada	**Area in EDs**: Management: decision making, resource allotment and ED discharge. **Location**: Canadian Journal of Emergency Medicine. **Methodology**: Design community service learning course: to form infographics established with content proficiency. **Problem/Issue**: To suggest a ground-breaking solution for less than 50% of emergency department patients who believed that discharge hand-outs conveyed health information effectively and even smaller number of patients believed that hand-out information would be helpful in care at home and to analyze the discharge sheets efficiency. **Visualization Kind**: Table and Figures. **Conclusion**: Clinician-patient debates will be simplified by information graphics for authorized decision-making; it will ease clinician-learner decisions established on proof-based guiding principles, and it will develop knowledge translation for health system managers and policy makers concerning suitable emergency department resource allotment. **Publication Kind**: Journal Article
Willinsky et al., 2016	Canada	**Area in EDs**: Management: Decision-Making; Intensive Care and Hospital Ward. **Location**: Canadian Journal of Emergency Medicine. **Methodology**: Qualitative: complete literature review of decision-making that took place from 1946 to 2015. **Problem/Issue**: To address decision-making for debilitated and overlooked patients in hospital situations. **Visualization Kind**: Table and Figures. **Conclusion**: There will be a vivid and dramatic increase in the number of patients as the Baby Boomers age. Articles identifying decision-making for debilitated and overlooked patients in the hospital situation. Decision-making procedures for debilitated and overlooked patients are explained by numerous articles none of which discuss ED. More investigation is required to find out the most proper and suitable technique of decision-making for patient unit in the ED. **Publication Kind**: Journal Article

(continued)

Table 3.2 (continued)

Author and year	Country	Extracted data
Lantz and Rosén, 2016	Sweden	**Area in EDs**: Management: Capacity of EDs and Operative Efficiency. **Location**: Journal of Health Organization and Management. **Methodology**: Queuing theory: arrival time, accurate time of triage and overall patients' number. Uses, arrival proportions and system capacity procedures to develop average queuing times. use the theoretical association among these three measures to develop system capacity measures depending on perceived arrival degrees and perceived average queuing times. **Problem/Issue**: To create a method depending on the queuing model for assessing the operational capacity in the service process without the process observation and utilize the technique for evaluating the operative capacity within the triage procedure. **Visualization Kind**: Mathematical Equations, Figures (Graph) and Tables. **Conclusion**: Hospital is trying to develop a progressive production and capacity planning system and is assessing effective capacity by using a trustworthy methodology. The queuing model is a feasible substitute for the traditional technique and direct observation. The technique is considered significant in assessing the effects of modifications in the work strategies and the staffing place. Management conclusions can be derived from the outcomes of the capacity approximations. **Publication Kind**: Research Paper
Donnelly, 2013	Canada	**Area in EDs**: Management: knowledge organization and patient documentation. **Location**: ProQuest LLC./Queen's University—Ontario. **Methodology**: Various techniques: case study, systematic scientific, systematic knowledge, and empirical observations. **Problem/Issue**: Use of secondary sources, such as continuing medical education (CME) and clinical practice guiding principle, to gather information on patients having various chronic disorders; crucial care physicians rarely gain access to the main sources of information. **Visualization Kind**: Tables and Graphs. **Conclusion**: According to the contemporary research, the subsequent policies and structures should have studied to encourage the arriving primary care workforce. All team members should receive training concerning the contribution of primary care and services to ensure that they get complete access to electronic health records to encourage both casual communication by means of the internal messaging features, formal patient documentation, and recommendations. **Publication Kind**: Thesis
Gautam, 2012	United States	**Area in EDs**: Knowledge Management—Health personal. **Location**: Minnesota State University. **Methodology**: Quantitative—A cross-sectional, descriptive, and correlational survey. **Problem/Issue**: To use the HBM model to reduce the frequency of disease. It has been one of the most frequently employed theories in health education and promotion. Health behaviour is decided by personal opinions or views on a certain disease and the existing approaches. **Visualization Kind**: Tables. **Conclusion**: Individuals will implement an innovative healthy behaviour or product if they believe they are vulnerable to a certain condition (heart disease), if they believe it will have possibly grave consequences, if they think that a guideline presented to them would be helpful in minimizing either their vulnerability or the seriousness of the condition. **Publication Kind**: Dissertation

(continued)

Table 3.2 (continued)

Author and year	Country	Extracted data
Chen et al., 2006	United States	**Area in EDs**: Management: decision support in triage room. **Location**: Physiological Measurements. **Methodology**: Mathematical modelling: for every sampled reference respiratory rate specific vital-sign monitor, quality index QI is measured by the algorithm. These data were gathered from patients in course of transport by the Life Flight helicopter service from the place of damage, 711 wounded patients were recorded and formulating and authorizing the qualification algorithm. **Problem/Issue**: To create a different group of automatic triages, diagnostic and prognostic algorithms that can help care providers make decisions during the pre-hospital care of trauma fatalities. **Visualization Kind**: Mathematical Equations, Figures, and Graph. **Conclusion**: For time series respiratory data, an automatic, quantitative respiratory data quality indexing system was created. The significance of the respiratory data qualification technique is supported by the research. The relationship developed between the physiological results and the respiratory data approach shows that care is required in choosing temporary data for algorithm development, which will predict clinical outcomes. **Publication Kind**: Journal Article
Van Geffen et al., 2016	Netherlands	**Area in EDs**: Management: Hospitalization: Bacterial and Infection Detection. **Location**: Journal of Breath Research. **Methodology**: Quantitative: preliminary study. **Problem/Issue**: To determine how an e-nose can be used as a screening device to discover bacterial and viral respiratory infections. To identify if participants have a bacterial, viral, or no respiratory tract infection. (Viral infections, Bacterial infections). **Visualization Kind**: Graphs and Table. **Conclusion**: The innovative screening device has proven to be an effective tool for identifying the absence or presence of a bacterial or viral infection. The breath of a sequence of well-diagnosed people as per the groups of the protocol decision requires to be taken concerning the existence of infection. All participants are part of the special interest group. **Publication Kind**: Journal Article
Teunissen et al., 2011	Netherlands	**Area in EDs**: Management: Patients Monitoring. **Location**: Journal of Physiological Measurement. **Methodology**: Experimental techniques: 0 heat flux technique. Every participant was told about the objective of the study, protocols, experimental processes and any related risks and profits before confirming their agreement to participate. **Problem/Issue**: To identify the performance of an innovative ZHF device on the forehead concerning these problems, to identify the performance of the new zero heat flux device with reference to the problems of short delay time, consistency, and non-intrusiveness. **Visualization Kind**: Table and Figures. **Conclusion**: The tool traced effectively with little to no time delay during stable, increasing and decreasing without wind and assessing better than the conventional rectal measurement. Hence, the ZHF technique can be implemented in practical situations. the ZHF sensor tracks oesophageal temperature in the stable and hot atmosphere, and it might be a feasible choice for the precise and non-intrusive estimation of temperature. **Publication Kind**: Journal Article

Table 3.3 Healthcare workforce

Author and year	Country	Extracted data
Allnutt et al., 2016	Canada	**Area in EDs**: Skills and Competencies. **Location**: Australian Health Review. **Methodology**: Quantitative (survey) study: information sheet and a consent form are sent to nurse practitioners who are supposed to employ five patients to take part in the study by means of a self-administered questionnaire. **Problem/Issue**: To assess the understanding of patients regarding the part played by the nurse practitioners (NP) and their contentment, quality of care, knowledge, and expertise. **Visualization Kind**: Tables. **Conclusion**: According to the findings, patients are only moderately aware of the role of the nurse practitioners. A broader awareness among community members regarding the role of NPs may help in increasing their positive impact on healthcare. **Publication Kind**: Journal Article
Flop, 2012	Australia	**Area in EDs**: Skills and Competencies. **Location**: Journal of Health Organization and Management. **Methodology**: Qualitative: interactive interviews to provide information regarding how leadership is explained by healthcare professionals. **Problem/Issue**: To assess the way the hybridity concept can help in re-theorizing leadership in the healthcare sector because it is linked to clinician managers (or hybrid-professional managers). Challenges the people formulating health reform policies concerning clinician manager's leadership programs. **Visualization Kind**: Tables. **Conclusion**: Novel methods are offered by hybridity to develop leadership programs and strategies in healthcare sector, which are uniquely positioned to deal with reform issues. **Publication Kind**: Journal Article
Rosenberg and Hickie, 2013	Australia	**Area in EDs**: Skills and Competencies. **Location**: Australian Health Review. **Methodology**: Qualitative: classification and reviewing. **Problem/Issue**: To allow the Independent Hospital Pricing Authority to comprehend the domain of mental health: where it is now by trying to use Activity-Based Funding (ABF) and to formulate and assess important and innovative models of care. **Visualization Kind**: Text: Percentages and Classifications. **Conclusion**: The activity-based funding (ABF) program has the potential to use preferred regulatory reasons to enhance further hospital-based facilities in the mental care division. **Publication Kind**: Journal Article

(continued)

Table 3.3 (continued)

Author and year	Country	Extracted data
Perry et al., 2014	United States	**Area in EDs**: Skills and Competences: health workforce and effectiveness. **Location**: Annual Review of Public Health. **Methodology**: Qualitative (classification): review. **Problem/Issue**: Evaluating how successful health programs are in the health of the general population. Several factors play a part in the health of populations, such as political, social, and economic factors, such as poverty and education levels. **Visualization Kind**: Tables and Charts. **Conclusion**: According to the research findings, when there is correct training, supervision, and allotment of the required medicines, equipment, and resources, community health workers can enhance critical behaviours and provide the necessary service accessibility. **Publication Kind**: Journal Article
Ricketts, 2011	United States	**Area in EDs**: Skills and Competences: workforce need and demand model. **Location**: Annual Review of Public Health. **Methodology**: Qualitative (review): ways of assessing health workforce distribution. Regression models for supply make use of time trends to forecast the upcoming supply of practitioners. **Problem/Issue**: To determine the number of people in a given population who may need a limited constellation of services, conforming to the requirements of an aging population with sufficiently proficient healthcare practitioners. **Visualization Kind**: Text: Percentages and Classifications. **Conclusion**: When the process is open, the best available data can be used to obtain feasible choices, and alternative situations would enable the policy makers to arrive at better planning decisions. There is insufficient expertise in the USA Healthcare workforce to fulfil the needs of an aging population. **Publication Kind**: Journal Article
Chartier et al., 2016b	Canada	**Area in EDs**: Skills and Competencies: quality improvement and patient safety. **Location**: Canadian Journal of Emergency Medicine. **Methodology**: Quantitative: a national multimodal needs assessment was developed, consisting of a survey. **Problem/Issue**: To explain the skills, stressing quality improvement and patient safety (QIPS). **Visualization Kind**: Figures. **Conclusion**: QIPS should be officially included in residency training. The study identified challenges, including the dearth of qualified and available faculty to develop and explain QIPS knowledge to residents, which demonstrated the need for a formal QIPS curriculum. **Publication Kind**: Journal Article

Table 3.4 Emergency preparedness

Author and year	Country	Extracted data
Baumgartner et al., 2008	United States	**Area in EDs**: Emergency Preparedness: risk factors associated with illness. **Location**: Wilderness and Environmental Medicine. **Methodology**: Quantitative Research: national hospital ambulatory medical care surveys. **Problem/Issue**: To collect information regarding the rates of occurrence and the risk factors related to hypothermia illness, i.e., low body temperature. **Visualization Kind**: Tables and Graphs. **Conclusion**: To decrease the occurrence of hypothermia in the community. Subsequent studies should concentrate on recognizing modifiable risk factors and formulating and applying strategies that specifically fulfil the requirements of vulnerable groups. **Publication Kind**: Journal Article
Clark, 2010	United States	**Area in EDs**: Emergency preparedness: emergency management operations. **Location**: ProQuest LLC./University of Baltimore-Maryland. **Methodology**: Mixed quantitative and qualitative assessment: data from one federal fiscal year 2008 (action research). **Problem/Issue**: To decrease risks and vulnerabilities that may lead to disasters, concentrating on the predominant national emergency management structure. **Visualization Kind**: Tables. **Conclusion**: Preparedness capability has led to a better understanding of emergency management organizations operations and has increased success with six interrelated components: command and management, preparedness, resource management, communication, and information management, supporting technologies, management, and maintenance. **Publication Kind**: Dissertation
Savkin et al., 2008	Russia	**Area in EDs**: Emergency preparedness: emergency response, operational intervention criteria and emergency regulation and guidelines. **Location**: Journal of Radiological Protection. **Methodology**: Mixed quantitative: and qualitative (classification): threat analysis of medical consequences. **Problem/Issue**: To recognize the radiological and medical factors pertinent to emergency response and readiness for medical emergency response at facilities to numerical variations in operational intervention criteria under situations that are otherwise identical. **Visualization Kind**: Tables and Math Equation. **Conclusion**: In Russia, emergency preparedness has been influenced considerably by the expertise in emergency response. In the widespread system of response pertinent to emergency preparedness, the medical and sanitary delivery of emergency response is given the highest priority. There is a special exercise pertaining to emergency regulations medical response at the site. After successful discussion between regulators, developers and operators, special regulatory guidance is given. **Publication Kind**: Research Paper

(continued)

Table 3.4 (continued)

Author and year	Country	Extracted data
Nikolai, 2014	United States	**Area in EDs**: Emergency preparedness: patient safety, risk management, and disaster response management. **Location**: Computer Science and Engineering- University of Notre Dame- Indiana. ProQuest LLC. **Methodology**: Mixed Quantitative: observation (gathered and examined key documents, including past situation reports, after action reports, and exercises documents.) and Qualitative (classification): informal and formal interviews for emergency managers. **Problem/Issue**: Crises involve coordinating new types of collective action and critical problem-solving in a particular situation. It requires the coming together of people, authorities, and resources in a particular period for a certain purpose. **Visualization Kind**: Tables and Charts. **Conclusion**: The study findings were significant for the study of emergency management and emergency processes. The simulator can help in training emergency personnel and in studying decision-making in emergency management. **Publication Kind**: Dissertation
Fridell and Ekberg, 2015	Sweden	**Area in EDs**: Emergency preparedness: safety in exposure to radiation. **Location**: Journal of Radiological Protection. **Methodology**: Qualitative studies- to create knowledge regarding the qualities or features of different events (focus group interviews and individual in-depth interviews). **Problem/Issue**: To obtain "as low as reasonably achievable" (ALARA) exposure to radiation. It is also critical to acknowledge the significance of protecting patients and themselves to ensure there are no long-term and short-term negative effects. **Visualization Kind**: Table and Figures. **Conclusion**: Much attention needs to be given to radiation protection issues in clinical management. This needs to be done in a transparent way and examples of the way the problem should be managed and prioritized are needed. **Publication Kind**: Journal Article

Table 3.5 Quality engineering

Author and year	Country	Extracted data
Nasr-Esfahani et al., 2016a	United States	**Area in EDs**: Engineering: Images (X-ray) Segmentation. **Location**: IEEE Engineering in Medicine and Biology Society. **Methodology**: Segmentation methods: neural network/deep learning; convolutional neural networks. These methods are grouped into three categories: tracking-based, model-based, and filter-based. **Problem/Issue**: To improve the quality of X-ray and explain vessel division in images that are normally of low quality and are suffering from noise for Coronary artery disease—the most widely prevalent heart disease. **Visualization Kind**: Figures. Tables and Mathematical equations. **Conclusion**: It is shown in the experimental findings of angiography images of a dataset that the suggested method performs better in extracting vessel regions. **Publication Kind**: Conference Paper
Nasr-Esfahani et al., 2016b	United States	**Area in EDs**: Engineering: Graphic Processing. **Location**: IEEE Engineering in Medicine and Biology Society. **Methodology**: Neural network: deep learning method. **Problem/Issue**: To help a dermatologist in diagnosing this kind of skin cancer in the early stages, i.e., skin-cancer-melanoma detection: the suggested mechanism employs clinical images. **Visualization Kind**: Figures, Tables, and Mathematical equations. **Conclusion**: It is demonstrated in the experimental findings that the suggested technique provides better diagnostic precision as compared to the state-of-the-art methods. **Publication Kind**: Conference Paper
Jafari et al., 2016	United States	**Area in EDs**: Engineering: images processing (Detection and diagnosing Skin Cancer) and feature extraction. **Location**: Annual International Conference of the IEEE Engineering in Medicine and Biology Society (EMBC). **Methodology**: Algorithms for digital images amplify the details and extract qualities to determine surface. **Problem/Issue**: It is suggested in the study that there should be efficient method for pre-screening the pigmented skin lesions. **Visualization Kind**: Graphs, Figures, and Mathematical equations. **Conclusion**: It was shown in the findings that the system could achieve a sensitivity of 90% compared to the latest techniques. There were very few omissions in identifying melanoma and the affected skin lesions. **Publication Kind**: Conference Paper

(continued)

Table 3.5 (continued)

Author and year	Country	Extracted data
Jamali et al., 2016	United States	**Area in EDs**: Engineering: Utilization of Patient's Record and Quality of Images. **Location**: Annual International Conference of the IEEE Engineering in Medicine and Biology Society (EMBC). **Methodology**: Experimental: robust watermark method- Advance image processing and diagnostic/ discrete Fourier transform. **Problem/Issue**: When used in the extraction stage of medical image, a robust watermarking technique is suggested in the study in which the watermark data is concealed in non-region of interests to avoid distortion of the region of interests. **Visualization Kind**: Graphs, Figures, and Mathematical equations. **Conclusion**: According to the experimental findings, the method is successful and provides better results in comparison to other similar methods. Watermarking framework was put forward to enhance robustness and to maintain the watermarked data's fidelity. The quality of the image and the watermark remains indiscernible. **Publication Kind**: Conference Paper
Kadkhodaei et al., 2016	United States	**Area in EDs**: Engineering: Quality—Automatic segmentation and Images processing. **Location**: Annual International Conference of the IEEE Engineering in Medicine and Biology Society. **Methodology**: Experimental-algorithm: the proposed technique performs better than the similar method to train a random decision forest that consists of different features obtained from detected volume of interest. The proposed method combines hybrid clustering and logistic regression. **Problem/Issue**: To facilitate an energy minimization problem, classify brain MR images. Classification forest was used to group the problem into a classification task with the help of various features extracted. In this study, automatic segmentation was used for the diagnosis. **Visualization Kind**: Graphs, Figures, and Mathematical equations. **Conclusion**: Artificial neural networks (ANN) are found to be robust computational models that are based on biological human neural mechanism. These networks use a group of effective features, and it is possible to train the neural network. **Publication Kind**: Conference Paper

Table 3.6 Utilization in healthcare

Author and year	Country	Extracted data
Morgans and Burgess, 2012	Australia	**Area in EDs**: Utilization: EDs, Ambulance and Measurements. **Location**: Australian Health Review. **Methodology**: Qualitative: Comprehensive Literature Review. **Problem/Issue**: To define and measure inappropriate emergency healthcare utilization and its impact on demand. **Visualization Kind**: Text: Percentages and classifications. **Conclusion** The examination of the meanings of 'Inappropriate' emergency healthcare utilization led to the recognition of two patient groups; emergency healthcare utilization by the people who are not facing a health emergency; and those are not seeking emergency healthcare, but they should. The literature review gives rise to questions regarding the patients' understanding of the part played by emergency healthcare services during an emergency. **Publication Kind**: Journal Article
Abourbih et al., 2016	Canada	**Area in EDs**: Utilization: ED resources—triage room. **Location**: Canadian Journal of Emergency Medicine. **Methodology**: Mixed Method: Observational Study, Phone Interviews and Control Group. **Problem/Issue**: To examine the availability of a triage tool in the subsequent follow up of concussion patients who have come to the emergency department and to make sure that the required actions are performed to deal with issues in the triage room. **Visualization Kind**: Tables and Graphs. **Conclusion**: It is important to have objective measures to find out if a system eventually decreases healthcare use for various healthcare resources. **Publication Kind**: Journal Article
Fauteux-Lamarre et al., 2016	Canada	**Area in EDs**: Utilization: Reduction of LOS. **Location**: Canadian Journal of Emergency Medicine. **Methodology**: Qualitative: Assessing a phenomenon: two groups of people that are assessing different outcomes are compared; the study is carried out on a smaller scale and can possibly cater to rare diseases that are similar to case-control study. The study included 274 patients from June 2012 to March 2014. **Problem/Issue**: To assess the effect of the Bier block on the hospital's duration of stay and the outcomes after the decrease of forearm fracture in contrast to the procedural sedation and to compare Bier block and procedural sedation to decrease forearm fracture. **Visualization Kind**: Tables. **Conclusion**: Bier block was related to a decreased emergency department duration of stay and lesser negative events, having no variations in reduction success or return visits. **Publication Kind**: Journal Article

(continued)

Table 3.6 (continued)

Author and year	Country	Extracted data
Yau et al., 2016	Canada	**Area in EDs**: Utilization: Healthcare Cost and Resources. **Location**: Canadian Journal of Emergency Medicine. **Methodology**: Qualitative: prospective cohort study—controlled group at four tertiary care EDs from Feb 2012 to Feb 2013 obtained patient demographics, medical history, 30-day SAE, EMS time points (call received, EMS arrival on scene, EMS departure from scene, time of transfer of care in the ED and ED duration of stay. **Problem/Issue**: To examine the patients shifted to ED by Emergency Medical services assessed a thirty-day serious negative event among the syncope patients shifted by the EMS. 66% are shifted to ED by Emergency Medical Services (EMS). **Visualization Kind**: Tables and Charts. **Conclusion**: A significant percentage of patients coming to the ED through EMS experience no serious adverse event (SAE) within 30 days, while 10.3% experience SAE within 30 days. Similarly, it was found in the study that there was a need to have an EMS clinical decision assistance to shift low-syncope patients to alternative care providers, like family physicians or rapid access clinics. When this tool is developed and executed, it has the potential to decrease EMS burden, ED crowding as well as healthcare costs. **Publication Kind**: Journal Article
Pandit, 2013	United States	**Area in EDs**: Utilization: Resource allocation optimization and real-time algorithm. **Location**: Computer Science—UNIVERSITY OF CALIFORNIA. ProQuest LLC. **Methodology**: Experimental: Webster's algorithm: real-time optimization methods—multi-user resource allocation (Content Aware Networking) adaptive Webster's method and simulation methodology. **Problem/Issue**: To find a delay-reducing minimizing cycle time or assessing delay for a cyclic, executed signal control system. Because of the existence of robust and inexpensive processing ability, the issue of resource allocation may be resolved through optimization techniques in real time. The OAF algorithm functions in the same way as the vehicle actuated traffic technique, yet it still generates lesser delays when compared with Webster's technique and pre-timed signal management. **Visualization Kind**: Graphs, Figures, and Mathematical equations. **Conclusion**: The vehicular traffic signal control application single-hop communication is enough and hence, we focused on explaining and characterizing the working of the physical layer and MAC layer protocols of IEEE. The WAVE protocol is used to allow the vehicular traffic scheduling algorithm and it was found that because of the kind of movement within city environments, bandwidth requirements would be less and would enable excellent grain horizons optimization communication. **Publication Kind**: Dissertation

Table 3.7 Simulation in healthcare

Author and year	Country	Extracted data
Russell et al., 2016	Canada	**Area in EDs**: Simulation: skills and knowledge. **Location**: Canadian Journal of Emergency Medicine. **Methodology**: Quantitative: national survey. **Problem/Issue**: To describe the use of simulation in Canada. **Visualization Kind**: Tables and Charts. **Conclusion**: Frequently used training modality. However, there is much variation in the structure, frequency, and timing of simulation exposure for residents. The shift to competency-based medical education requires a national standardized approach. **Publication Kind**: Journal Article
Cheung, 2011	United States	**Area in EDs**: Simulation: geometric optimization, algorithm simulate the process, minimized process, and algorithm approximation. **Location**: Faculty of Computer Science, University of Texas at Dallas. ProQuest LLC. **Methodology**: Algorithm simulates the process. **Problem/Issue**: Three geometric optimization issues are considered, which include a weighted polygonal subdivision R in the space or plane. Shortest path problem with obstacles. Geometric problems: to change the problem and make its representation natural or simpler, allowing us to view the problem from a unique perspective. **Visualization Kind**: Figures and Math Equation. **Conclusion**: The shortest path problem in R3 with obstructions. Two approximation algorithms are presented for the point-to-face shortest path problem in R3. The point-to-face shortest path can be approximated by positioning a group of Steiner points on the target face. In future studies, the approximate shortest path between geometric objects may be calculated, such as edges, faces, polytopes, etc. in R3. It was demonstrated in the study that every problem version could be reduced to a certain optimization process that may be resolved by calculating the polynomials roots or algorithms approximation. **Publication Kind**: Dissertation

were suggested. Significant associations among the different contexts of healthcare systems throughout Canada [26, 28, 31, 36] and the USA were shown by the data mining procedure and suitable dynamic actions were recommended. In [18] E-Health was found to support the reengineering business model of healthcare provision. Similarly, in [46], the reengineering model showed the excellence of care obtained. In [26], learner proximity was found to be an important factor affecting the documentation and evaluation of medication implementation using the described tools.

A healthcare organization operates according to its management, which is applicable to all kinds of organizations, including businesses, governmental organizations, and non-profit organizations. Management focuses on accomplishing the aims and objectives of the organization by including various human, financial, natural, and technological resources. Management is the heartbeat of an organization because it connects all the departments. When there are poor managerial skills in an organization, the organizational performance is low [62]. An critical area of EDs and hospital functionality in general is time management [36]. In ED, triaging process should be eliminated, and three different types of international scales used in the process (CTAS), (ESI) and (ATS). The patient spends time in the waiting area, in visiting the doctor, in the consultation room, in laboratories, and in queues [45]. The ED is sometimes unable to offer medical care to patients in a timely manner, which may be life-changing because it may lead to unwarranted injuries, pain, or untimely death.

Time refers to ticking of the clock, seconds, minutes, hours, days, years, and seasons. This is the literal meaning of time, but a patient who is waiting for a doctor feels quite differently about time compared to a person who is enjoying its passage. Patients who are waiting may feel frustrated, and time becomes magnified because of the pain, anxiety, and inactivity that they are experiencing while they wait. In addition, patients may benefit greatly from a discussion about their health [42], which may have a considerable, positive impact on their diagnosis. As a result of the discussion, the patient might have gained confidence and courage in undergoing treatment successfully. Because health facilities have insufficient funds, EDs are usually crowded, which leads to personal risk [62]. Nonetheless, the management can reduce overcrowding by making efficient [15] use of the physicians and nurses that are available [37].

There has been a rapid increase in the use of wireless technology because of the advancements in technology and the extensive use of mobile phones. Wireless technology [16] is also used to a significant extent in maintaining health because it helps in allocating resources [43] more efficiently. Technology plays a key role because it helps to reduce the amount of time spent in seeking the doctor, including waiting time, consultation, diagnosis, and possibly the time spent in undergoing laboratory tests and obtaining medicines. Technology makes possible the automatic uploading of data with no involvement by the user. The individual identifier is private, and the long-term medical records of patients are maintained [16]. Nonetheless, it should be pointed out that the non-performance of weak governments brought about the active adoption of mHealth [16] facilities to decrease costs. MHealth [17] employs internet-based technology in which a mobile phone is used to monitor a person's health. Various applications, such as steps analyzers, real motion assistances, cerebral health trackers, and other analytical systems that employ real-time data, are installed for this purpose.

The term competency refers to the potential of a person to complete a task in an efficient and effective manner based on the knowledge, capability, and expertise of the person. The term skills refers to the potential of a person to perform a task expertly and competently compared to other people. Although there are different definitions of skills and competencies [8, 9], the terms can be used interchangeably. Specialists in different fields are competent and skilled enough to better manage the prevailing issues compared to other people. Examples are doctors, electricians, teachers, and psychologists. These people have the skills required to perform the tasks better than an ordinary individual could.

Many differences exist in the way health services are provided in communities [8] with respect to the availability and quality of critical health care. The government provides funds to public hospitals; however, service delivery in these hospitals lags behind private hospitals in terms of resources, missions, and operations. The performance of a public health facility [25] is mainly dependent on the way its resources are organized. It is not easy for hospitals to retain competent practitioners, which influences their capability to improve their performance.

The greatest disadvantage of a group is inadequate trust among its members. Other related disadvantages are disagreement, insufficient sense of responsibility, avoidance of accountability, and neglecting the results when one member prioritizes individual needs rather than the collective objectives [65]. Tutoring helps to achieve the highest potential of team members, which can be done by recognizing queries, providing answers, emphasizing limitations, supervising individual relationships, and fostering inherent capabilities. Maximizing the potential of team members would lead to the creation of healthy groups and the reduction in group failure, conflict, and damage [66]. Better performance can result from mixed or shared systems compared to centralized or decentralized systems. The former systems employ their resources to the highest degree because they are flexible in meeting the requirements of the community.

The issue of emergency preparedness [53] has raised the awareness of safety as a vital issue in any situation. Moreover, it has key role in encouraging discussions between the regulators, designers, and operators that are involved in the process with stringent adherence to the established regulatory frameworks. Because of the increased number of hypothermia complications, research should focus on recognizing the risk factors [21] that may be altered easily to suit the context. In addition, the process requires the adoption of strategies that cater to the requirements of vulnerable groups. An equal part in fulfilling safety requirements is played by the medical response to emergencies [61]. The need for preparedness in managing emergencies raises questions about the part played by safety providers in this process [56, 59]. There should be a sufficient supply of medical and sanitary equipment. An alternate emergency preparedness technique is to have additional personnel at hand who are vigilant to deal with any emergency whenever it arises [61].

Several engineers are worried about dealing with image segmentation [47] as observed in the workings of X-ray machines. Excellent performance has been achieved in the experiments with angiography when mining for vessel sections. It has been found that these regions show segmented images which are most likely not relevant for medical explanations. In addition, the dermatologists consider it relevant to use graphic processing [48], applied using a neural network to determine skin complications. The process is considered accurate, and it is highly pertinent in comparing findings.

An experimental-algorithm approach has been used in the diagnosis process to determine automatic segmentation [51] and image processing. It is found in the study that automatic glioma tumors segmentation is a diagnostic tool. The process consists of computational models [49] that can present effective features, which improve the diagnostic procedure.

The assessment of the study on the basis of the concept of EDs utilizations involved theoretical hierarchies. Various studies have been conducted by different authors, pertaining to the utilization in the healthcare sector, which has led to the development of concepts for their assessment. Following these studies, different conclusions and deductions have been reached with respect to the issue of EDs utilization. Therefore, in this study, utilization in the healthcare sector has been explained as a significant approach in EDs, particularly with respect to healthcare cost [39] and resource allocation with the help of real-time algorithm [57].

The most significant issue examined in EDs utilization was the description and the measurement [11] of the inappropriate utilization of the emergency health and its effect on the demand. The result assessment included the text made up of the percentages and the classifications. Following the assessment of the definitions of the inappropriate use of the emergency healthcare, two classes [34] of patient cohorts were recognized. The first kind involved the utilization of emergency healthcare by those patients who were not experiencing health emergency, and the other kind was the group that requires emergency healthcare but does not seek it. Additional research can be carried out on how the patients comprehend the role of services in the emergency healthcare [22].

In the studies performed in Canada on the use of simulation that on average, the students performed 20 h of a simulation exercise [41]. It was claimed by majority of the students that the time spent on simulation training was sufficient to fulfill their needs. In addition, it was stressed by most of the respondents that there was inter-professional interference in the simulation. For geometric optimization issues [52] that have a weighted geometric border in the space, the shortest path problem in space permits the approximation of the point-to-face of the smallest path using the location of a point on the target face. This method may be used to address issues in EDs, such as the transport of patients by ambulance.

3.1 RQ1: Which Techniques Were Used in the ED Research?

The response to this question was divided into seven parts that were mainly obtained from tables, as demonstrated in Fig. 3.6. The different methods shown in each section have been used in these fields. Our findings showed that almost nine distinct techniques were employed in the research on EDs. Efficiency factors in quality care were examined using qualitative, meta-analysis systematic reviews to obtain information. Mixed methods research was used to obtain results regarding issues that were pertinent to management and to determine the causes of the quality issue. Quantitative studies often collect longitudinal data. However, in the research on emergency care operational management, five distinct methods were used. The occurrences of each technique were as follows. Regarding the qualitative method, the systematic review of the literature helps in analyzing data, demonstrating significant results. The idea of time in EDs was analyzed and the results were used to formulate a fixed system and address decision-making settings in EDs and hospitals. Quantitative methods also help to determine allocative efficiency, compare spending with patient outcomes, and to compare EDs.

In addition, quantitative methods are used to describe ED patients and to examine the tools created by ED personnel. Experimental methods also help in defining triage room utilization in the ED setting and to conduct rapid analyses with the help of experimental techniques. There was limited use of the mixed methods technique. The evidence obtained through the mathematical modeling approach was used to formulate and verify decision support with the help of algorithm (real-time) or queuing theory to examine operation ability. In the section pertaining to workforce skills and competencies to explain competencies while stressing quality, quantitative and qualitative methods were used to examine and assess effectiveness and to enhance improvement. Quantitative approaches were used in emergency preparedness studies to review and examine the risk factors related to illness. However, to decrease hazards, the mixed methods technique allows for the coordination of new kinds of collective actions and the enhancement of effectiveness. In addition, simulation was found to affect operation management. Engineering quality, such as X-ray segmentation and graphic processing, require computational techniques such as algorithms and neural network (deep learning) to determine failure with a possibility of 90%. The utilization and simulation in the health care sector were shown by algorithms that processing time was decreased.

3.2 RQ2: Which Themes Were Introduced in the ED Research?

The selected themes were grouped based on ED research topics. The EDs activities were explained properly. Mapping was used to explain the main issues in EDs and the techniques employed to study them [9–27]. These were not affected by a particular topic. Therefore, the limitations of the research were recognized in terms of emergency preparedness, healthcare quality, performance measurement, patient satisfaction, and the healthcare industry, as shown Figs. 1.3 and 1.4.

3.3 RQ3: When and Where Was the Research Published?

Several journals issued between the years 2010 and 2017 were included in each database. The earliest study was published in 1864. There was an increase in the importance of this field between 2010 and 2014, which was followed by a significant decline in 2017. The present study considered only peer-reviewed journals, materials, and conferences to answer the research question. The percentages of the articles according to theme are shown in Figs. 3.3 and 3.4. The studies on engineering, simulation and process management constituted only 2% of the total studies on EDs published from 2010 to 2017.

3.4 RQ4: How Did the Research Illustrate the Results?

The methods used to illustrate the results in the research are shown in Tables 3.1, 3.2, 3.3, 3.4, 3.5, 3.6 and 3.7. The results were usually shown in graphs, figures, and tables.

3.5 RQ5: What Problems Were Addressed in the Research?

In some emergency management, the dynamic and iterative procedures that reduce risks and exposures may be unregulated. In healthcare systems, active and repetitive procedures, such as parallel computing, dissemination, exchanges, and the unethical application of correct knowledge can lower the quality of service or lead to incorrect crisis management. In crisis management, simulation, focus, exceptions, memory, authorities, people, and resources must be created simultaneously at a specific time and for a specific purpose. ED issues can be grouped into significant concerns, as shown in Tables 3.1, 3.2, 3.3, 3.4, 3.5, 3.6 and 3.7 and in Figs. 3.1, 3.2 and 3.6. Examining and describing new measurements supported the assessment of how patients are affected in the triage room. Optimization and real-time algorithms helped in identifying delays in cycle time and decreasing ED processes to improve the ability of resource allocation. Process time was decreased to reduce the patient pathway, which could be optimized when simulations and real-time algorithms were used in EDs (Figs. 3.3 and 3.4).

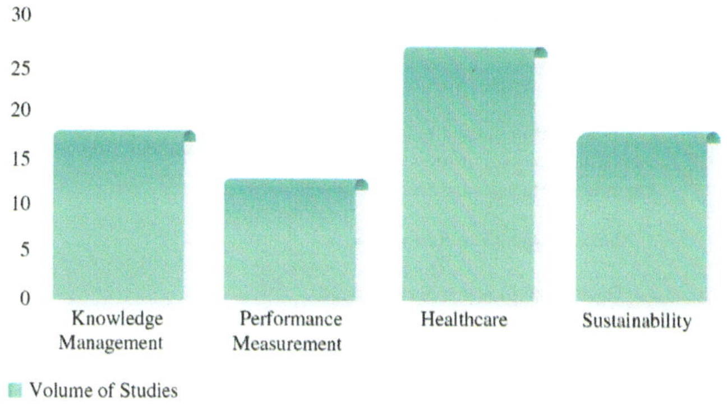

Fig. 3.1 Subjects with a research gap in performance measurement

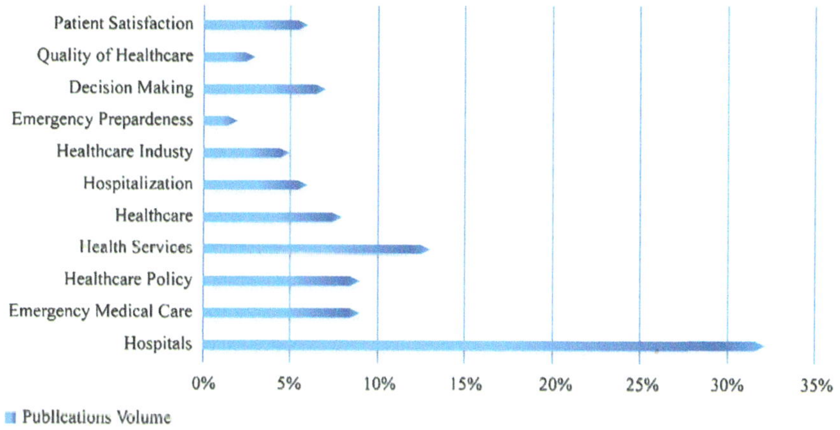

Fig. 3.2 Overview of topics with research gaps (emergency preparedness and quality of healthcare)

3.6 RQ6: How Was the Research Classified?

The classification of the research is shown in Fig. 3.5. Figure 3.6 provides an overview of the systemic clustering that was developed using the taxonomy of the content described in Tables 3.1, 3.2, 3.3, 3.4, 3.5, 3.6 and 3.7. Figures 3.5 and 3.6 show the classifications of quality of care, workforce competencies and skills, emergency care management, emergency preparedness, quality engineering, utilization, and simulation in EDs. In addition, when the contents of the selected studies was classified, it was revealed that the number of reviews was limited. Therefore, further systematic mapping and systematic review studies are needed (Table 3.8).

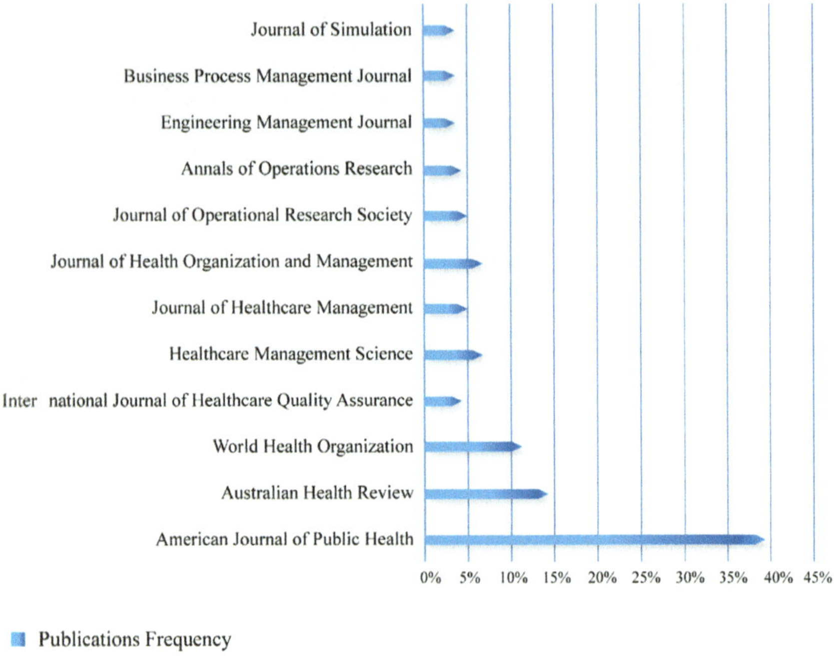

Fig. 3.3 Where the studies were published

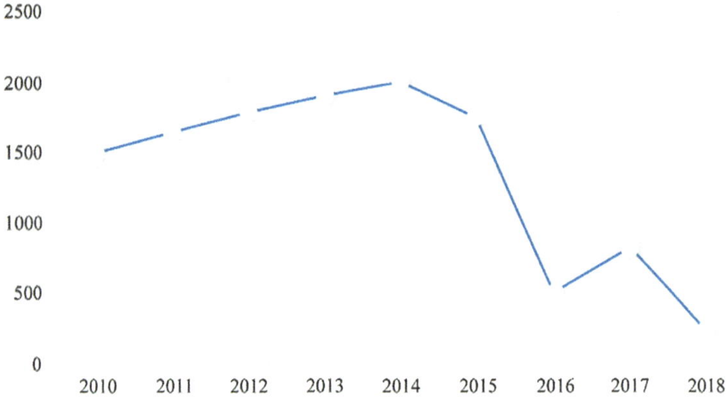

Fig. 3.4 When the studies were published

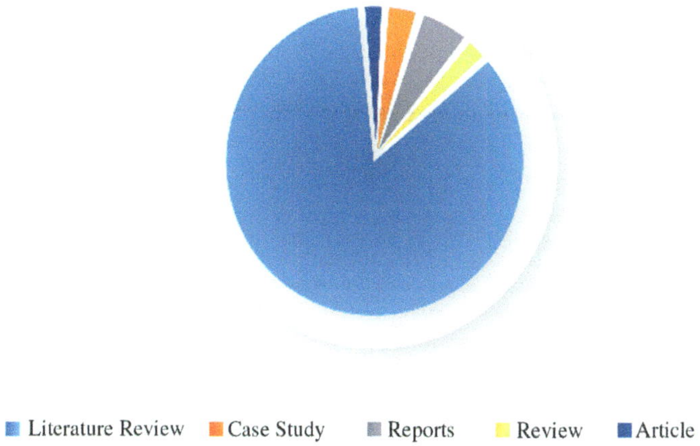

Fig. 3.5 Classification of studies

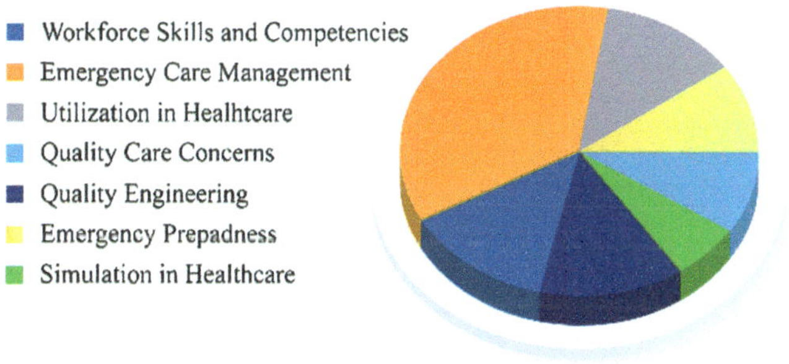

Fig. 3.6 Thematic studies cluster

Table 3.8 Thematic clusters with references

Theme name	References number and occurrence
Quality care	[13, 14, 18, 16, 28, 31, 36, 46]
EDs operational management	[10, 15–17, 23, 24, 27, 29, 30, 32, 33, 35, 37, 38, 40, 42–45, 54, 55, 58, 60, 62]
Healthcare workforce	[8, 9, 12, 17, 20, 25]
Emergency preparedness	[21, 53, 61, 56, 59]
Quality engineering	[47–51]
Utilization in healthcare	[11, 22, 34, 39, 57]
Simulation in healthcare	[41, 52]

Chapter 4
Discussion

Table 3.1 presents the findings of our systematic review study regarding quality care, general and present concerns. Several significant quality concerns pertaining to healthcare emerged in the findings, particularly in EDs; however, in this study, these concerns were restricted to significant areas deemed important by any quality EDs seeker. Careful management is required in quality care [63]. Hence, the foremost priority in healthcare systems is management, that is, to describe, measure, assess, enhance, and regulate service quality by utilizing a step-by-step increase in the ability of EDs from incomplete service processing to high-quality procedures and hence to optimal outcomes [64]. Other management trends included patient classification [32], patient diagnosis, common symptoms [14], which require electronic patient records. Patient records [14, 28] are integral with cloud computing [18] solutions and data warehousing to increase the potential of data mining techniques [2] to predict ability and obtain significant and usable information.

In addition, cloud computing solutions [18] play a valuable role in assisting performance analyses [26] with the help of documentation. Furthermore, seekers of quality care should concentrate on process improvement and continuous quality improvement [46] using modern techniques and process reengineering [36, 46]. Nonetheless, skills and competencies [31] need to be implemented to enhance performance. Figure 4.1 shows a classification tree of quality care that is part of groups and subgroups with the focus on management's continuous quality improvement and e-health.

The emergency care management model can significantly affect the patient pathway. Patient-centered care comprises listening to, informing, and considering patients. Hence, in offering respectable and responsive care according individual patient preferences, requirements, and values, relevant clinical decisions prioritize the patient. In addition, in patient-focused care, services are decentralized. Services consist of inputs that perform processing simultaneously to offer sufficient care. For instance, the input-process-output (IPO) can be carried out by computer [64], as shown in Fig. 4.2. Hence, simulation is used in various situations to prepare patients in the normal zone or the hazard zone.

S. Ben Zayed et al., *System Reengineering in Healthcare: Application for Hospital Emergency Departments*, Studies in Systems, Decision and Control 172,
https://doi.org/10.1007/978-3-319-98104-8_4

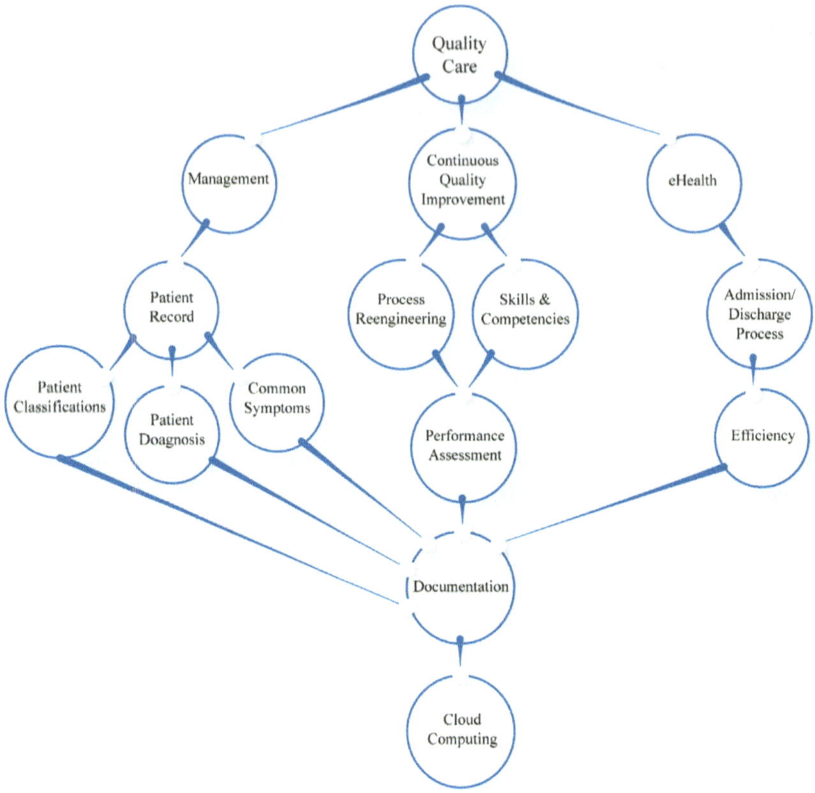

Fig. 4.1 Quality clusters in healthcare

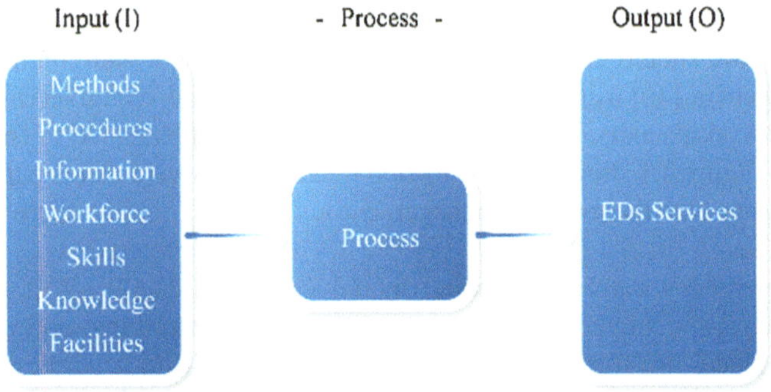

Fig. 4.2 Input-process-output (IPO) model

Figure 4.2 shows that services need to be based on modern management. Hence, the electronic information flow in the ED system is the first step. Overcrowding in EDs [27] was linked to EDs capacity [45] as well as the healthcare workforce.

These factors are related, and further studies need to be carried out to determine the case mix in EDs [29]. Figure 4.2 summarizes the information presented in Table 3.2 and serves as a guideline for EDs future managers of EDs. The guideline should be followed to enhance patient satisfaction [40] and the overall patient outcomes of care services [37]. Seven areas were identified, which were considered the major areas of the study of ED management: structured strategies, quality tools, triage level, mhealth, knowledge management, patient focus, and ambulance service. These findings indicate that the areas that are significant in the daily operations of EDs require skilled people to serve as managers. A background in medicine should not be a requirement. Instead, these managers should have backgrounds in engineering or in contemporary applied management. It is very important to spend time with a patient [23] instead of staring at computer screens and noting the negative points of the patient's illness. Doctors should avoid asking negative questions about the patient's mistakes or anxieties. Instead they should converse with the patient and try to help them heal psychologically before taking any medicines. This consideration would make the patient feel respected and that no resources are wasted. In the healthcare sector, doctors should not serve as managers at any level.

Mobile electronic [17] machines have already profoundly affected capacity developments in medicine. A significant part can be played by technology in developing an effective system that ensures suitable end-of-life care. The concept lattice that demonstrates the significance of technology in the field of medicine is described below.

Overcrowding continues to be a problem in EDs. As explained earlier, managers of health centers should ensure the maximum utilization [42] of physicians and nurses. The patients who are in the most critical condition should be treated first. This point is important: several deaths and life-changing conditions are caused by delays in treatment. Managers should also ensure that the ED is large enough to reduce overcrowding and ensure optimal air circulation. There should also be the maximum utilization of technology to maintain records of every patient's treatment history. Placebos should still be used by doctors and nurses in the rapid treatment of a patient because some people need motivation and support in having a positive attitude toward the medical process [44]. The classification tree of emergency care operational management cluster is demonstrated in Fig. 4.3, which is divided into groups and subgroups. The figure shows the structure strategies, EDs ambulance, mHealth, triage room, quality standardized tool, patient focus, and knowledge management in a contemporary EDs management operation real-time monitoring system.

Healthcare practitioners [20] should have the skills and competencies required to meet the needs of the elderly population. As Figs. 4.3 and 4.4 show, the most important issues concern the way in which public hospitals function, which is why their performance differs from that of private hospitals. Public health services should benefit from the resources provided by the government to offer improved healthcare services to patients. The grantees should alter their conditions to allow health care facilities to carry out research to improve emergency care. This should also be considered an initiative for other stakeholders to prioritize the health of the community to which they provide services. Based on this kind of motivation, there would be a

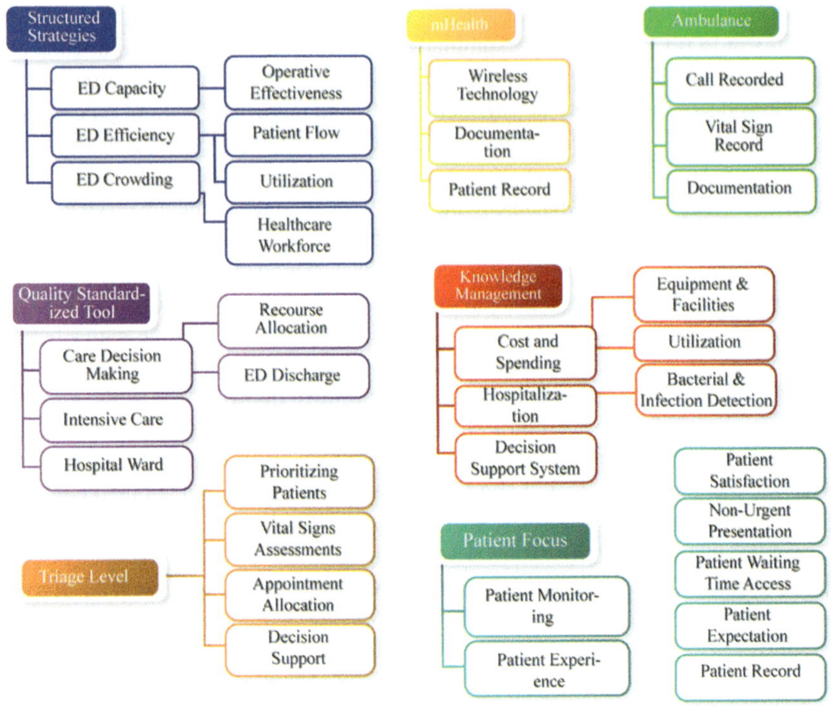

Fig. 4.3 EDs operational management cluster

substantial improvement in the healthcare performance of public hospitals. When suitable training [25], supervision [19], selection and delivery of the required medication, equipment, and resources are in place, then an important role can be played by community health [18, 19] workers to enhance the critical behavior and provide access to the required services. The techniques used to improve the performance of the health workforce should initially concentrate on the existing staff to avoid spending time in training new staff. By implementing a hybrid program, it would be possible to achieve significant enhancements rapidly with respect to the availability, proficiency, responsiveness, and efficiency of healthcare workers by using various low-cost and practical tools and by developing leadership to enhance healthcare techniques [9]. Figure 4.4 illustrates the classification tree of workforce competencies and skills, which is divided into groups and subgroups. The focus is on knowledge versus skills.

Figure 4.5 shows a significantly enhanced model of the performance of healthcare workers [67].

The experience of emergency response has considerably influenced emergency preparedness [61]. The medical and sanitary delivery of emergency responses is a significant activity in the widespread system of actions pertaining to emergency

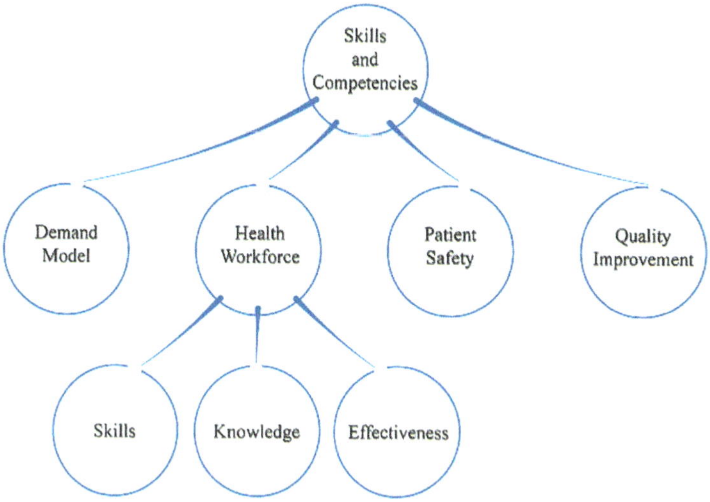

Fig. 4.4 Workforce clusters in healthcare

preparedness. Medical response at the site is regulated by activity that is specific to emergencies. Substantial attention needs to be paid to issues of disaster operational management by medical management. This process should be transparent, and it should serve as an example of how the problem should be managed by allotting it the highest priority. Health challenges [21], risks, and vulnerabilities have been recognized as augmenting the difficulties that are commonly faced in dealing with emergencies. Consequently, a significant part has been played by appropriate emergency preparedness in comprehending and developing working command and operational management systems [53], scales of preparedness, resource utilization to achieve these goals, communication and information management, delivery of the required technology [56], and using related maintenance and management systems.

Figure 4.6 shows the classification tree of emergency preparedness in the healthcare sector, which is divided into groups and subgroups. As Fig. 4.6 shows, the mainstream emergency preparedness concentrates on the management of EDs from the operational management perspective, in which safety is the prevailing issue in addition to emergency regulations and directives. Hence, it is important to perform simulation and practice activities to develop a disaster response program in the hazard mode [53] and to ensure that the functions of EDs in the normal mode are efficient and effective. The process will comprise training in simulation, improving research-based approaches, and using the required equipment to support the functions. A significant role is played by simulation in ensuring the safety of a society that may be influenced by radiation, floods, and other such events. In this process, the most critical aspects are problem-solving and the prioritization [52] of needs. Hazards [41] that may lead to a disaster can be decreased by developing a national emergency management system.

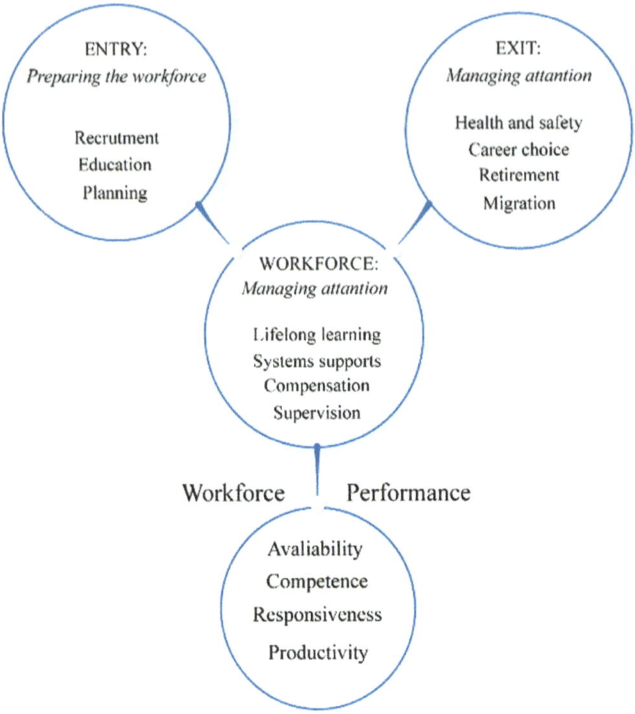

Fig. 4.5 Healthcare workforce performance model

Eventually, the goal is to develop a mutual understanding of the prescribed procedure in the quality engineering of EDs. The digital imaging [49] (i.e., the magnification of the subject's details) offers a 90% sensitivity to skin infections and cancer. In contrast to the other techniques, digital imaging has been observed to lower the occurrence of errors and the lapses in identifying melanoma and other skin lesions.

The classification of quality engineering is shown in Fig. 4.7, which is divided into groups and subgroups of streams focusing on quality engineering in healthcare. The use of patient records [50] and the quality of images in analysis have improved prescription procedures. These improvements have been supported by the development of placing a watermarking technique on the image to provide security to the most critical part of the image. This method has been shown to improve the robustness and fidelity of the data. In addition, it has been noted that watermarked data were secured from being noticed by non-experts who may have negative intentions. In contrast to other methods, this method provided improved outcomes.

The utilization of EDs was studied by examining their resources [22], which include the triage room. Future research should be conducted to determine whether the triaging tool helps in the ensuing follow up of concussion patients who have come to the emergency department and to ensure that the relevant steps are taken to

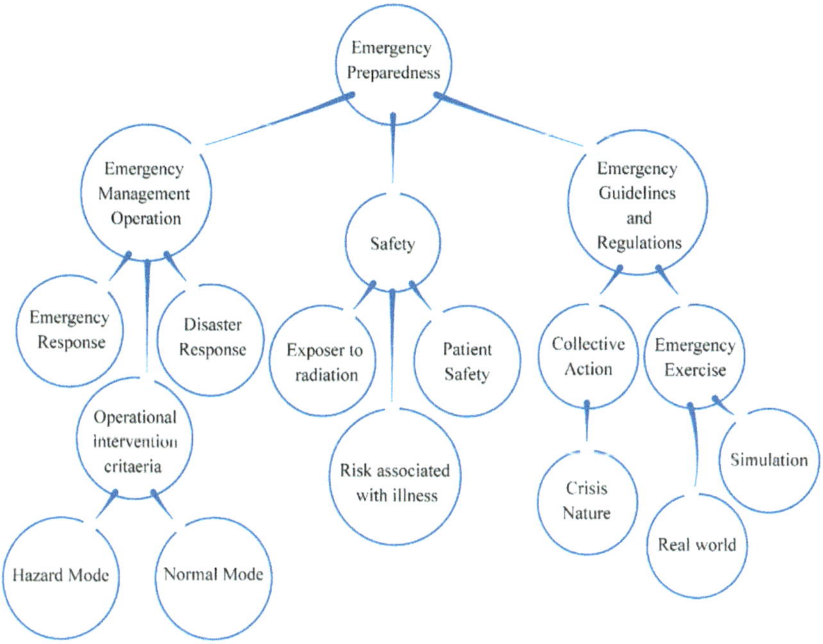

Fig. 4.6 Emergency preparedness clusters in healthcare

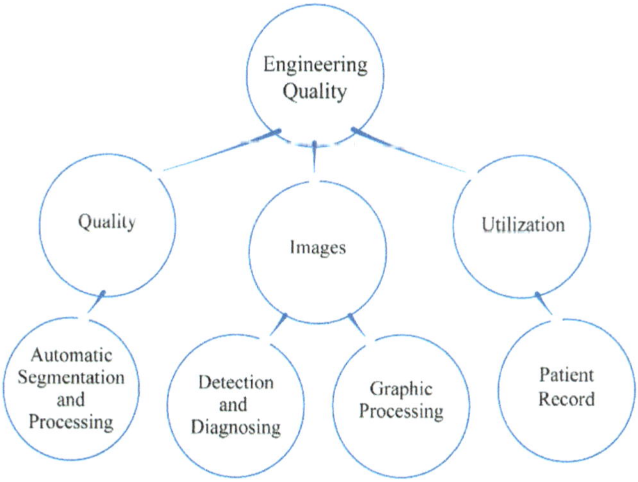

Fig. 4.7 Quality engineering clusters in healthcare

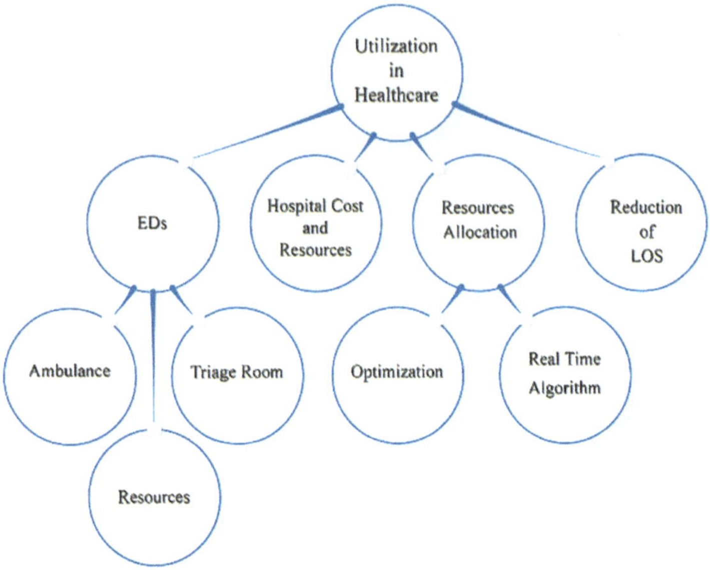

Fig. 4.8 Utilization clusters in healthcare

deal with problems in the triage room. It was recommended that objective measures should be applied to determine whether the system eventually reduces the utilization of different healthcare resources.

The qualitative research approach was used to perform analyses of the utilization of EDs, ambulances [11] and the measurements. Using this approach, an extensive literature review was performed. The examination of the descriptions of the inappropriate use of emergency healthcare revealed two kinds of patient groups. In the first group, emergency healthcare was used by patients who did not require emergency treatment. The second group included patients that did not use emergency healthcare even though they required emergency services. It is recommended that objective measures be applied to determine whether the system eventually leads to the lower utilization of healthcare for different healthcare resources and to ascertain that adequate actions are taken to solve the issues in the triage room. A decrease in the LOS [34] in EDs with less negative effects decreased health costs. Figure 4.8 demonstrates the classification tree of the utilization of healthcare services. The focus is on resource allocation through the use of real-time algorithms and decreased LOS and operational expenses in healthcare.

Resource allocation [57] and the optimization of the real-time algorithm were examined using an experimental research technique that consisted of Webster's algorithm, the real-time optimization model, and multi-user resource allocation. The author wanted to determine the delay time in a decreased cycle and to assess the delay in the executed cyclic signals and control systems. For instance, the control

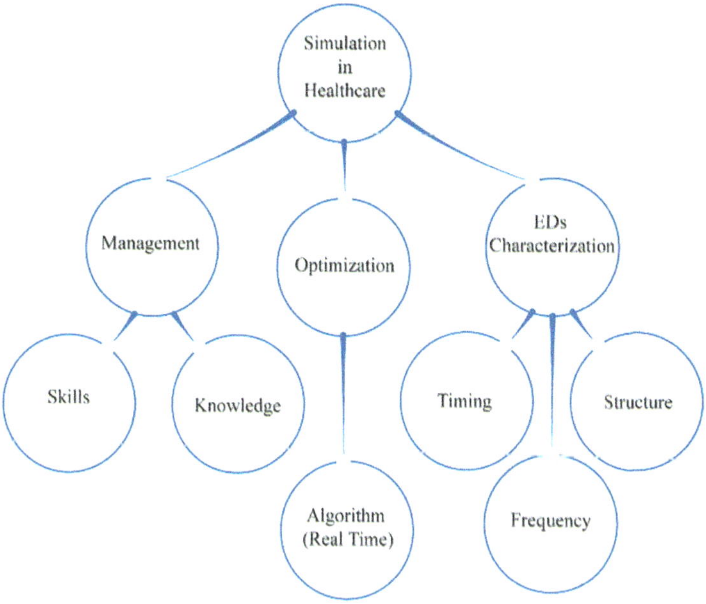

Fig. 4.9 Simulation clusters in healthcare

application of the vehicular traffic signal provides "single-hop" communication in a suitable and corresponding manner.

Figure 4.9 shows the classification tree of simulations in healthcare. The tree is divided into groups and subgroups. The focus is on the simulation of the entire system, comprising management, optimization, and ED characterization. This simulation involves the structure and organization of EDs, the frequency of patients (i.e., patient flow), and the timing of processes, such as admission time, LOS, and discharge. In addition to the real-time algorithm, skills and expertise are required to apply the simulation and to decrease the outcomes of healthcare procedures.

Simulation-based activities are significant features of medical residency programs [41]. There is a certain degree of variability in the ways in which simulation-based activities and other related activities are carried out; however, the objective of these programs is to raise competency levels in medical education. Hence, it is critical to determine the variabilities that exist and to review them with regard to the impact on the competency levels in the residency programs in Canada. The results of this study were shown to be valid and reliable. It is possible to reproduce the study to determine whether the results can be generalized or to assess whether there have been any significant variations in the structure of simulation-based education. In [52], a novel method was used to solve simulation issues, which was precise in generating simulation outcomes.

Chapter 5
Conclusion and Future Research Directions

5.1 Conclusion

Emergency management involves several complex factors. An analytical decision-making process should be used to assess a health technology based on its performance. It is important to update this analytical system frequently because modeling processes are important in managing patient and staff communications as well as patient care systems in hospitals. This finding is significant because the ED and the problems that surface in the ED are complex. Various studies have used mathematical models. However, only a few studies have applied mathematical models to ED systems. The results of these studies are critical because they could lead to decreasing wait times in EDs. Important issues and methods were obtained from mapping the research, which helped in obtaining solutions [2]. A few mapping studies are being carried out at present [7]; however, very few studies are focusing on EDs [18–21]. The vital areas that should be analyzed concern the quality of the study selection and the continuous updating of research [8]. The findings of the present mapping study demonstrated the dynamic issues in EDs as well as the methods used to address these issues and obtain positive results.

In developing countries, the healthcare systems are severely lacking in patient services. Therefore, it is crucial to address the outstanding issues and meet the requirements for critical hospital-based healthcare. The implementation risks of activity-based funding also need to be managed. Based on the findings of this study, the following solutions are recommended: continuous training and simulations are needed by emergency preparedness systems as well as comprehensive information analyses. Evidence-based practice (EBP) in EDs and its effective and efficient inclusion in clinical and managerial leadership continues to be a challenge. It is necessary to utilize a structure, framework, process, and outcomes based on scientific classification to determine the existing obstacles to the adoption of EBP.

S. Ben Zayed et al., *System Reengineering in Healthcare: Application for Hospital Emergency Departments*, Studies in Systems, Decision and Control 172,
https://doi.org/10.1007/978-3-319-98104-8_5

The main factors are the people, authorities, and assets involved in managing an emergency. The focus should be on patients' experiences, satisfaction levels, successful processes, patient security, and rapid response programs. An experienced operational management team that has knowledge, skills, and experience in quality improvement, modeling, simulation, and process reengineering should oversee the operation of EDs and the processes involved. Hence, a greater number of doctors should perform their job as doctors instead of managing tasks and procedures within the healthcare system, particularly in EDs. Therefore, to manage healthcare personnel and its service delivery, it is critical that engineers with a background in lean six-sigma and quality assurance are on the management team. In this study, the classification trees developed for quality care, ED operational management, workforce competencies and skills, emergency preparedness, engineering quality, utilization and simulation in healthcare explain the given terms as parts of EDs even though ED is the whole and explaining each term for its classification tree refers to parts.

With regard to simulation modeling in EDs, the current situation as well as the shortcomings in the previous research should be examined [7]. It is important to conduct multi-label case studies of healthcare workers to identify workforce competency with respect to skills and abilities [30]. Leadership [10] within management [28] is required in EDs to ensure that control is maintained [29]. It is important to manage EDs and impart knowledge to personnel while considering EDs' policies, capacity, structure, network, and so on to ensure that there is informed decision-making, the successful operational management of emergency cases in normal and disaster situations, and less crowding and more regulation in EDs. Emergency processes will be applied efficiently when the methods have been evaluated and the appropriate one has been practiced.

5.2 Future Research Direction

The findings of this systematic review study could be used to update the standards of healthcare quality. The research that should be performed in the future with respect to emergency and risk management is shown in Fig. 3.3 [31]. Because the present study was conducted to offer short-term results similar to [8], the findings should be considered preliminary. Future studies should focus on the sustainability of executing real-time data monitoring in EDs, the performance measurement of emergency mechanisms in EDs, the operational management of EDs, process reengineering in EDs, and the use of simulation in EDs. Furthermore, emergency preparedness, patient satisfaction, waiting time and overcrowding with patient experience; problems, challenges and solutions national studies from operational research prospective shall be conducted and reported in the near future along with healthcare workforce skills and competencies national study.

References

1. Petersen K, Vakkalanka S, Kuzniarz L. Guidelines for conducting systematic mapping studies in software engineering: an update. Inf. Softw. Technol. 2015; 64:1–18
2. Almozayen NA, Othman MKB, Gani AB, Alharethi SZ. Data mining techniques: a systematic mapping review. In: Saeed F, Gazem N, Patnaik S, Saed Balaid A, Mohammed F, editors. Recent trends in information and communication technology. IRICT 2017. Lecture notes on data engineering and communications technologies. Cham: Springer; 2018.
3. Alharethi S, Bin Gani A, Bin Othman M. Emergency departments: a systematic mapping review. Future of information and communications conference (FICC) 2018. Singapore: IEEE Signal Processing Society; 2018
4. Lim M, Nye T, Bowen J, Hurley J, Goeree R, Tarride J. Mathematical modeling: the case of emergency department waiting times. Int J Technol Assess Healthc. 2012;28(02):93–109.
5. Gul M, Guneri A. A comprehensive review of emergency department simulation applications for normal and disaster conditions. Comput Ind Eng. 2015;83:327–44.
6. Elberzhager F, Münch J, Nha V. A systematic mapping study on the combination of static and dynamic quality assurance techniques. Inf Softw Technol. 2012;54(1):1–15.
7. Paz F, Pow-Sang J. A systematic mapping review of usability evaluation methods for software development process. Int J Softw Eng Appl. 2016;10(1):165–78.
8. Allnutt J, Allnutt N, McMaster R, O'Connell J, Middleton S, Hillege S, et al. Clients' understanding of the role of nurse practitioners. Aust Health Rev. 2010;34:59–65.
9. Flop L. Leadership, clinician managers and a thing called "hybridity". J Health Organ Manage. 2012;26(5):578–604.
10. Hanson R. Good health information—an asset not a burden! Aust Health Rev. 2011;35(1):9.
11. Morgans A, Burgess S. Judging a patient's decision to seek emergency healthcare: clues for managing increasing patient demand. Aust Health Rev. 2012;36(1):110.
12. Rosenberg S, Hickie I. Making activity-based funding work for mental health. Aust Health Rev. 2013;37(3):277.
13. Scott I. Preventing the rebound: improving care transition in hospital discharge processes. Aust Health Rev. 2010;34(4):445.
14. Abrahm J. Advances in palliative medicine and end-of-life care. Annu Rev Med. 2011;62:99–187.
15. Baicker K, Chandra A, Skinner J. Saving money or just saving lives? Improving the productivity of US healthcare spending. Annu Rev Econ. 2012;4(1):33–56.
16. Clifford G, Clifton D. Wireless technology in disease management and medicine. Annu Rev Med. 2012;63(1):479–92.

S. Ben Zayed et al., *System Reengineering in Healthcare: Application for Hospital Emergency Departments*, Studies in Systems, Decision and Control 172,
https://doi.org/10.1007/978-3-319-98104-8

17. Kaplan R, Stone A. Bringing the laboratory and clinic to the community: mobile technologies for health promotion and disease prevention. Annu Rev Psychol. 2013;64 (1):471–98.
18. Meier C, Fitzgerald M, Smith J. eHealth: extending, enhancing, and evolving healthcare. Annu Rev Biomed Eng. 2013;15(1):359–82.
19. Perry H, Zulliger R, Rogers M. Community health workers in low-, middle-, and high-income countries: an overview of their history, recent evolution, and current effectiveness. Annu Rev Public Health. 2014;35(1):399–421.
20. Ricketts T. The healthcare workforce: will it be ready as the boomers age? A review of how we can know (or not know) the answer. Annu Rev Public Health. 2011;32(1):417–30.
21. Baumgartner E, Belson M, Rubin C, Patel M. Hypothermia and other cold-related morbidity emergency department visits: United States, 1995–2004. Wilderness Environ Med. 2008;19 (4):233.
22. Abourbih D, Bedi S, Hunt C, Ouchterlony D, Ackery A. P001: Concussion patients in the emergency department: assessing a new triaging tool for follow-up and prompt long term management. CJEM. 2016;18(S1):S79.
23. Atkinson P. What then is time? An exploration of time perception in emergency medicine. CJEM. 2016;18(04):293–5.
24. Chartier L, Bosco L, Lapointe-Shaw L, Chenkin J. Use of point-of-care ultrasound in long bone fractures: a systematic review and meta-analysis. CJEM. 2016;19(02):131–42.
25. Chartier L, Vaillancourt S, McGowan M, Dainty K, Cheng A. LO093: A national needs assessment survey for the development of a quality improvement and patient safety curriculum for Canadian emergency medicine residents. CJEM. 2016;18(S1):S62.
26. Cheung W, Dudek N, Wood T, Frank J. LO080: Performance and proximity: exploring resident factors that impact the quality of work-based assessments. CJEM. 2016;18(S1):S57–8.
27. Ducharme J. Healthcare in Canada—where? when? for whom? CJEM. 2016;18(02):133–5.
28. Grafstein E, Sharma D, Aggarwal V, Innes G, Stenstrom R. P049: A novel administrative database solution for capturing ED patient co-morbidity—the derived Charlson Comorbidity Index. CJEM. 2016;18(S1):S95.
29. Holroyd B, Rosychuk R, Jelinski S, Bullard M, McCabe C, Rowe B, et al. P063: Is triage score a valid measure of emergency department case mix? CJEM. 2016;18(S1):S99–100.
30. Imperato J, Mehegan T, Henning D, Patrick J, Bushey C, Setnik G, et al. Can an emergency department clinical "triggers" program based on abnormal vital signs improve patient outcomes? Corrigendum. CJEM. 2016;19(01):80.
31. Jensen J, Travers A. Contemporary evidence-based practice in Canadian emergency medical services: a vision for integrating evidence into clinical and policy decision-making. CJEM. 2016;19(03):220–9.
32. Krebs L, Chetram R, Kirkland S, Nikel T, Voaklander B, Davidson A, et al. LO091: Non-urgent presentations to the emergency department: patients' reasons for presentation. CJEM. 2016;18(S1):S61.
33. Krebs L, Villa-Roel C, Ospina M, Holroyd B, Rowe B. P068: Developing a standardized knowledge dissemination tool for communicating the need for Choosing Wisely© in Alberta's emergency departments. CJEM. 2016;18(S1):S101.
34. Fauteux-Lamarre E, Burstein B, Cheng A, Bretholz A. Reduced length of stay and adverse events using bier block for forearm fracture reduction in the pediatric emergency department. Pediatric Emergency Care. 2016:1.
35. Leggatt L, Davis M, Columbus M, McGuire J, Spadafora A. P079: Comparison of vital sign documentation for pre-hospital "lift-assist" calls and non "lift-assist" calls. CJEM. 2016;18 (S1):S105.
36. Leung A, Duic M, Gao D, Whatley S. PL003: Impact of process improvements on measures of emergency department efficiency. CJEM. 2016;18(S1):S29–30.
37. Leung A, Gong Z, Chen B, Duic M. LO009: Impact of physician navigators on measures of emergency department efficiency. CJEM. 2016;18(S1):S33.

38. MacKay J, Atkinson P, Howlett M, Palmer E, Fraser J, Vaillancourt E. P084: Waiting makes me sick: is it time for formal triage in primary care? CJEM. 2016;18(S1):S106.
39. Yau L, Mukarram M, Kim S, Arcot K, Thavorn K, Taljaard M, et al. LO083: Outcomes and resource utilization among syncope patients transported by emergency medical services. CJEM. 2016;18(S1):S58–9.
40. Pinto F, B-Lajoie M. P105: Patient outcome feedback in emergency medicine. CJEM. 2016;18(S1):S113.
41. Russell E, Hall A, Hagel C, Petrosoniak A, Dagnone J, Howes D. Simulation in Canadian postgraduate emergency medicine training—a national survey. CJEM. 2017:1–10.
42. Calder-Sprackman S, Kwok E, Bradley R, Landreville J, Calder L. P019: Understanding patient perceptions of emergency department wait time publication: a mixed-methods needs assessment. CJEM. 2016;18(S1):S84.
43. VandenBerg S, Ruhl G, Lang E. P137: Emergency department discharge information sheets—a prescription for success? CJEM. 2016;18(S1):S123–4.
44. Willinsky J, Hyun I. P140: Emergency department decision-making for incapacitated and unrepresented patients: a comprehensive review of the literature. CJEM. 2016;18(S1):S124–5.
45. Lantz B, Rosén P. Measuring effective capacity in an emergency department. J Health Organ Manag. 2016;30(1):73–84.
46. Buttigieg S, Gauci D, Dey P. Continuous quality improvement in a Maltese hospital using logical framework analysis. J Health Organ Manag. 2016;30(7):1026–46.
47. Nasr-Esfahani E, Samavi S, Karimi N, Soroushmehr SR, Ward K, Jafari MH, Felfeliyan B, Nallamothu B, Najarian K. Vessel extraction in X-ray angiograms using deep learning. In: 2016 IEEE 38th annual international conference of the Engineering in Medicine and Biology Society (EMBC); 2016 Aug 16. IEEE; 2016. p. 643–6.
48. Nasr-Esfahani E, Samavi S, Karimi N, Soroushmehr SM, Jafari MH, Ward K, Najarian K. Melanoma detection by analysis of clinical images using convolutional neural network. In: 2016 IEEE 38th annual international conference of the Engineering in Medicine and Biology Society (EMBC); 2016 Aug 16. IEEE; 2016. p. 1373–6.
49. Jafari MH, Samavi S, Karimi N, Soroushmehr SM, Ward K, Najarian K. Automatic detection of melanoma using broad extraction of features from digital images. In: 2016 IEEE 38th annual international conference of the Engineering in Medicine and Biology Society (EMBC); 2016 Aug 16. IEEE; 2016. p. 1357–60.
50. Jamali M, Samavi S, Karimi N, Soroushmehr SM, Ward K, Najarian K. Robust watermarking in non-ROI of medical images based on DCT-DWT. In: 2016 IEEE 38th annual international conference of the Engineering in Medicine and Biology Society (EMBC); 2016 Aug 16. IEEE; 2016. p. 1200–3.
51. Kadkhodaei M, Samavi S, Karimi N, Mohaghegh H, Soroushmehr SM, Ward K, All A, Najarian K. Automatic segmentation of multimodal brain tumor images based on classification of super-voxels. In: 2016 IEEE 38th annual international conference of the Engineering in Medicine and Biology Society (EMBC); 2016 Aug 16. IEEE; 2016. p. 5945–8.
52. Cheung Y. Optimization problems in weighted regions [PhD dissertation]. The University of Texas at Dallas; 2011.
53. Clark L. Implementation of national incident management system in New Jersey [PhD dissertation]. Baltimore, MD: University of Baltimore; 2010.
54. Donnelly C. Evaluation as a mechanism for integrated knowledge translation [PhD dissertation]. Kingston, ON, Canada: Queen's University; 2013.
55. Gautam Y. A study of assessing knowledge and health beliefs about cardiovascular disease among selected undergraduate university students using health belief model [PhD dissertation]. Carbondale: Southern Illinois University; 2012.
56. Nikolai C. SIMEOC: A virtual emergency operations center (VEOC) simulator for training and research [PhD dissertation]. IN: Notre Dame University; 2014.
57. Pandit K. Real-time resource allocation and optimization in wireless networks [PhD dissertation]. University of California Davis; 2017.

58. Chen L, McKenna T, Reisner A, Reifman J. Algorithms to qualify respiratory data collected during the transport of trauma patients. Physiol Meas. 2006;27(9):797–816.
59. Fridell K, Ekberg J. Making the invisible visible: a qualitative study of the values, attitudes and norms of radiologists relating to radiation safety. J Radiol Prot. 2016;36(2):200–14.
60. Van Geffen W, Bruins M, Kerstjens H. Diagnosing viral and bacterial respiratory infections in acute COPD exacerbations by an electronic nose: a pilot study. J Breath Res. 2016;10 (3):036001.
61. Savkin M, Sneve M, Grachev M, Frolov G, Shinkarev S, Jaworska A. Medical and radiological aspects of emergency preparedness and response at SevRAO facilities. J Radiol Prot. 2008;28(4):499–509.
62. Teunissen L, Klewer J, de Haan A, de Koning J, Daanen H. Non-invasive continuous core temperature measurement by zero heat flux. Physiol Meas. 2011;32(5):559–70.
63. Alharthi S. Offshore, outsourcing for information system projects, need carful management. Res J Sci IT Manag. 2017;02(11):20–6.
64. Alharthi S. Towards a sustainable competitive advantage. Int J Bus Res Dev. 2012;1(1).
65. Lencioni P. The five dysfunctions of a team. 1st ed. San Francisco: Jossey-Bass A Wiley Imprint; 2002.
66. Alharthi S. Forming, measuring, optimizing, human capital with enhancement concerning dynamic capability: update on theoretical framework. Res J Sci IT Manage. 2016;06(02):8–30.
67. WHO. The World Health Report. 2006: working together for health [Internet]. Who.int. 2017. http://www.who.int/whr/2006/en/. Accessed 22 Nov 2017.
68. NVivo QSR International. 55 Cambridge Street Burlington, MA 01803 USA: QSR International; 2017.

About the Authors

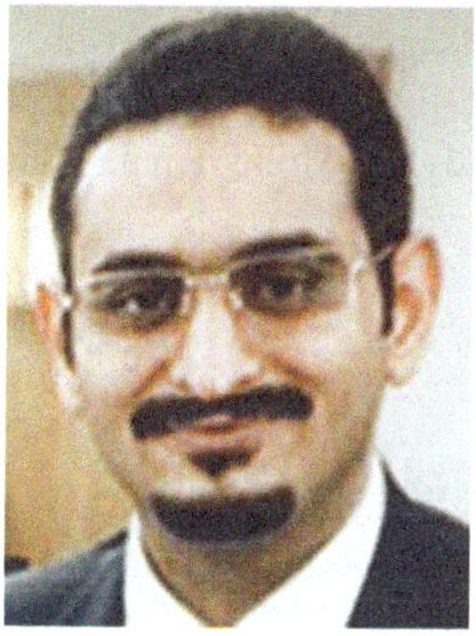

Eng. Salman Ben Zayed
Department of Computer System & Technology
Faculty of Computer Science & Information Technology (FSKTM)
University of Malaya (UM)

- Ph.D. Candidate and Certified International.
- Modeling and Simulation Expert.
- Lecturer & Associated Engineer at University of Umm Al-Qura.
- Lean Healthcare Advisor and Certified Kaizen Facilitator.
- Certified Lean Six Sigma and Six Sigma Master Black Belt.

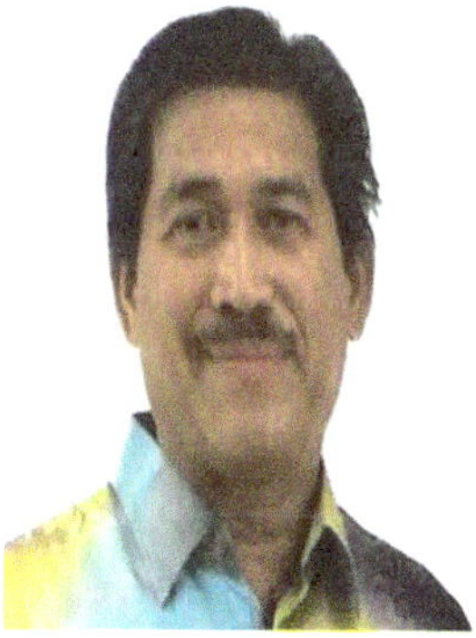

Prof. Dr. Abdullah Bin Gani
Department of Computer System & Technology
Faculty of Computer Science & Information Technology (FSKTM)
University of Malaya (UM)

- Senior IEEE member.
- Academy of Sciences Malaysia, Fellow.
- Mobile Cloud Computing Expert.
- Director of Mobile and Cloud Computing Centre—UM.
- Consultant and visiting professor to many universities.

S. Ben Zayed et al., *System Reengineering in Healthcare: Application for Hospital Emergency Departments*, Studies in Systems, Decision and Control 172,
https://doi.org/10.1007/978-3-319-98104-8

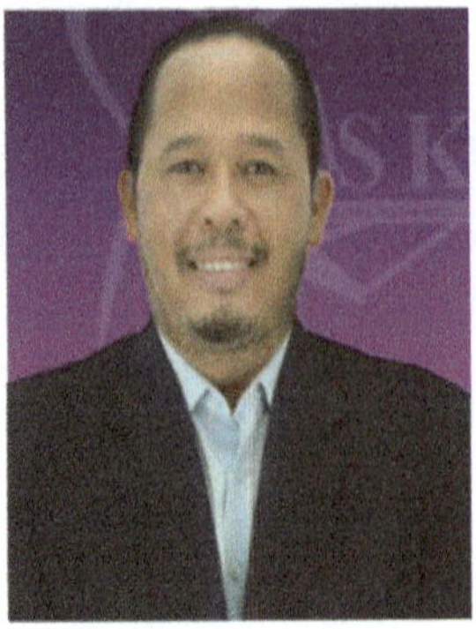

Dr. Mohd Khalit Bin Othman
Department Of Information System
Faculty of Computer Science & Information Technology (FSKTM)
University of Malaya (UM)

- Analysis of Algorithms and Complexity Expert.
- Business Intelligence Services Expert.
- Health Information Services Expert.
- Collaborative Computing Services and ICT Expert.

Corresponding Authors Emails: Eng.Salman Ben Zayed szharthi@uqu.edu.sa, Prof. Dr. Abdullah Bin Gani abdullah@um.edu.my and Dr. Mohd Khalit Bin Othman mkhalit@um.edu.my

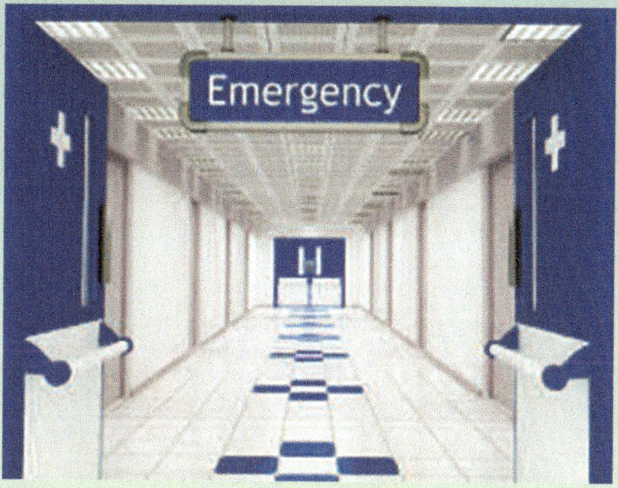

SPRINGER
NATURE

2018

The manufacturer's authorised representative in the EU is Springer Nature Customer Service Centre GmbH, Europaplatz 3, 69115 Heidelberg, Germany. If you have any concerns regarding our products, please contact ProductSafety@springernature.com

Printed and bound by CPI Group (UK) Ltd, Croydon, CR0 4YY
30/09/2026
02225664-0002